Unvaxxed

**The Crikey.
Read**

Unvaxxed

Trust, truth and the rise of vaccine outrage

DYANI LEWIS

Hardie Grant

BOOKS

Published in 2022 by Hardie Grant Books,
an imprint of Hardie Grant Publishing

Hardie Grant Books (Melbourne)
Wurundjeri Country
Building 1, 658 Church Street
Richmond, Victoria 3121

Hardie Grant Books (London)
5th & 6th Floors
52–54 Southwark Street
London SE1 1UN

hardiegrantbooks.com

All rights reserved. No part of this publication may be reproduced, stored in a retrieval system or transmitted in any form by any means, electronic, mechanical, photocopying, recording or otherwise, without the prior written permission of the publishers and copyright holders.

The moral rights of the author have been asserted.

Copyright text © Dyani Lewis 2022

 A catalogue record for this book is available from the National Library of Australia

Unvaxxed
ISBN 978 1 74379 882 9

10 9 8 7 6 5 4 3 2 1

Cover design by Josh Durham/Design by Committee
Typeset in Adobe Caslon Pro by Cannon Typesetting
Cover art based on *The Creation of Adam* by Michelangelo (1475–1564)

Printed in Australia by Griffin Press, part of Ovato, an Accredited ISO AS/NZS 14001 Environmental Management System printer.

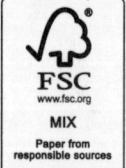 The paper this book is printed on is certified against the Forest Stewardship Council® Standards. Griffin Press holds chain of custody certification SGSHK-COC-005088. FSC® promotes environmentally responsible, socially beneficial and economically viable management of the world's forests.

Hardie Grant acknowledges the Traditional Owners of the country on which we work, the Wurundjeri people of the Kulin nation and the Gadigal people of the Eora nation, and recognises their continuing connection to the land, waters and culture. We pay our respects to their Elders past and present.

CONTENTS

Introduction	1
1. Unvaxxed or anti-vax?	15
2. Mistrust and the roots of (dis)belief	27
3. Networks of harm	39
4. Bad actors	53
5. An attempt to swindle nature	63
6. My body, my choice	77
7. Sowing divisions	89
8. What next?	99
Acknowledgements	116
Notes	119

INTRODUCTION

On 28 March 2020, the Facebook Messenger app on my phone pinged with a message from Mum. Forwarded from whoever had sent it to her, the message laid out some 'important information about the new coronavirus'. It should have been the first Saturday of school holidays for my eldest daughter, who had just started her first year of school. Instead, the term had ended early and abruptly. International travel was banned, gatherings were curtailed, and two days earlier, my home state of Victoria had recorded its first death from COVID-19. The world was on edge. I was on edge.

'The virus hates heat,' the message from Mum said, 'therefore hot drinks such as infusions, broths or simply hot water should be consumed abundantly during the day. Avoid drinking ice water or drinks with ice cubes.' It went on: 'For those who can, sunbathe. The Sun's UV rays kill the virus and the vitamin D is good for you.' According to the poorly punctuated, copy-pasted screed, the advice was originally sent as an internal email to staff at the Royal Brisbane Hospital. 'Please share with family, friends and work colleagues,' it implored. My mother diligently forwarded a second, abridged version of the same message, a moment after the first. It claimed to be 'SERIOUSLY EXCELLENT ADVICE by Japanese doctors treating COVID-19 patients'. It was obvious that neither claim was true and, to me at least, that the advice was nonsense.

'Unfortunately this is total BS,' I replied. 'Happy to talk – have spent last few days talking to experts on transmission.' Hot water won't stop the virus, I told her. Washing your hands is a good idea, I said. And facemasks make a difference, I added, even though not everyone was convinced of that at the time.

A couple of days later, Mum sent links to sewing patterns for facemasks, no doubt discovered on the same platform she'd found the other dubious messages. But a month after that, she sent me a video on YouTube. 'Have a look at this – really interesting!' she texted. The video was a webinar by Andrew Kaufman, a psychiatrist based in Syracuse, New York state. After reeling off his credentials, Kaufman laid out his thoughts on 'What I think COVID-19 really is'. Instead of being caused by a novel virus, Kaufman speculated, COVID-19 was probably caused by some other form of cellular assault – stress, perhaps, or a toxin – which was causing microscopic vesicles with a virus-like appearance under the microscope to form inside a person's lung tissue. Or maybe – though he couldn't find anything in the literature to support his theory – electromagnetic radiation from 5G mobile phone towers was the culprit. And those first cases of COVID-19 in the Wuhan wet market? Probably just a case of bad seafood, he said.

I called Mum straightaway. The doctor – who has since disavowed mainstream medicine – doesn't know what he's talking about, I said. I was terse as I invoked conspiracy theories and the stupidity of people to believe such garbage. Mum bristled and became defensive at my tone. 'OK, well I don't know. That's why I'm asking,' she said. I wonder whether even then, she was deciding to be more careful about what she shared with me.

Despite reporting on little else, I barely spoke of the pandemic with my mum over the next year or more. My world contracted around me. Lockdowns, home-schooling, and interviews about contact tracing, facemasks and specks of contagion carried on air currents dominated my days. But my mum's life away from Melbourne proceeded relatively untouched by COVID-19, which is not to say she wasn't dealing with other upheavals. A few months before the pandemic arrived on Australia's doorstep, she sold her house in the leafy hills of Melbourne's outskirts and temporarily moved in with her sister in Adelaide. Then, at the end of 2020 – having spent all of five days in lockdown – she moved again, this time to Canberra, to be closer to my brother and his kids, and to start afresh. Two weeks before Christmas 2020, they signed a lease together.

In August 2021, Canberra was on the precipice of its first lockdown when my brother texted me. 'So I'm kind of worried about [Mum]. She's gone [off] the deep end with covid conspiracies,' he wrote. 'Anti lock down, anti vaccine … all the right-wing loopy stuff from the states,' he wrote. His main concern was for his kids – aged eleven and nine at the time – who were being fed a diet of fearful warnings from their grandmother. Microsoft founder Bill Gates is bankrolling vaccine development, she told them, and they're not really vaccines at all, because they alter your DNA.

Her messages at the start of the pandemic suggested she had already tapped into some questionable networks online. But I'd ignored those crimson-bright warning signs. YouTube and Facebook algorithms – combined with her own tendencies to mistrust Western medicine and government authorities – had taken her to the darker corners of pandemic denial and conspiracy.

I was aghast and outraged on my brother's behalf. But I wasn't surprised. For as long as I can remember, my mum has held unconventional views. Mine was a homebirth. On a frosty Canberra morning, I slid into the world in the bedroom of a suburban weatherboard, midwife in attendance, oxygen tank at the ready. I received no childhood vaccines until I attended high school, and I was wholly unfamiliar with the idea of a family doctor. Mum was an acupuncturist and Chinese herbalist long before she qualified as a psychologist. And on repeated occasions she has demonstrated what I eventually saw as her credulous side – buying into cult-like religious groups and get-rich-quick schemes that inevitably failed or, more often than not, left her worse off than before.

I'd rarely challenged my mother on her beliefs. Perhaps out of cowardice, perhaps because of a sense that such efforts would be futile. Sometimes there were disquieting kernels of 'truthiness' in what she said; other times it was pure bunk. Either way, I'd had no interest in disabusing her of her passionately held sense that she'd discovered something of genuine importance.

A week later, my brother contacted me again. Mum had sent him a link to a YouTube video, 'MASS PSYCHOSIS – How an Entire Population Becomes MENTALLY ILL', which cunningly portrays the COVID-19 pandemic as an episode of propaganda-induced society-wide madness, à la the seventeenth-century Salem witch trials in Massachusetts, without ever mentioning the pandemic specifically. My brother tried to tell Mum that the science about the pandemic was conclusive. 'Bullshit,' she replied. 'It's not really about the science but what is being allowed to be reported.'

I shouldn't have taken it personally, but this hit a nerve. For eighteen months, COVID-19 had consumed my life both personally and professionally. And now my own mother was questioning the veracity of my work, not to mention my mental grasp on reality. I was incensed that she was painting me, a member of the media, as a dupe, wilfully doing the bidding of a power-hungry government, or worse, the money-grubbing corporations that make up 'Big Pharma'.

I called her, told her we were concerned. But there was little concern in my voice as I berated her for getting all her information from Facebook and YouTube. She started telling me about how fear-mongering propaganda can cause mass, population-wide psychosis. Then she turned to defending herself against my attack. Eventually, she just hung up.

In the weeks that followed, she launched a campaign to convince me that truth was on her side, that I was the one who was mistaken. With the vaccine rollout now in full swing around the country, she was determined to persuade me that the vaccines were dangerous. She'd send a video link. I'd reply with another link to debunk the video's content or expose the liars in the video who were peddling mistruths. 'If you believe in smear campaigns without knowing both sides that's fine. Can't believe you are so gullible,' she wrote. 'This is a repeat of the things that happened in Nazi Germany. The propaganda is unreal. But then telling you that is pointless so just forget it. No need to reply.'

As countries struggled to staunch the spread of COVID-19 in 2020, progress during that first pandemic year towards an effective vaccine was nothing short of extraordinary. 'A freaking miracle' is how health journalist Helen Branswell described it on the health news site *STAT* in February 2022. Just sixty-three days after the sequence of the SARS-CoV-2 virus was published, scientists were already injecting doses of Moderna's Spikevax into the arms of volunteers. That was on 16 March 2020, four days before Australia closed its international borders to non-citizens and non-residents arriving from overseas and the day Australia diagnosed its 401st case of COVID-19.

The speed of vaccine development outstripped all expectations. In February 2020, the World Health Organization (WHO) predicted that vaccine development would take at least eighteen months. Instead, it took less than a year. On 2 December, the United Kingdom became the first country in the world to authorise a COVID-19 vaccine when its Medicines and Healthcare products Regulatory Agency (MHRA) gave temporary regulatory approval for Comirnaty, the mRNA vaccine developed by German biotechnology company BioNTech and Pfizer, the American pharmaceutical behemoth.

The previous record-holder for vaccine development was Mumpsvax, developed by the prolific vaccinologist Maurice Hilleman, who worked for the American-owned Merck & Co. From the time Hilleman swabbed the throat of his sick daughter Jeryl Lynn in 1963 to collect a sample of the mumps virus, until the vaccine was approved by the US Food and Drug Administration, just four years elapsed.

Scientific triumph has come with a sting in its tail. Segments of the public have been alarmed by the speed of vaccine discovery and the novel technologies in the most widely injected vaccines available. An undercurrent of mistrust in the multinational pharmaceutical companies who developed the vaccines and the government agencies that fast-tracked their approval has fanned scepticism of the vaccines and the motives of those promoting them. The close ties between pharmaceutical companies, governments and scientific advisers have more than a whiff of impropriety about them. The upshot: people who have never before refused vaccines have now became staunch opponents to the COVID-19 jabs.

I'm far from alone in having a significant personal relationship catastrophically rupture over questions of how the pandemic has been managed, and over the COVID-19 vaccines in particular. Ask anyone, and they will tell you of a person in their orbit – a family friend, a brother-in-law, a colleague at work – who has chosen not to be vaccinated, lost their job because of vaccine mandates, or joined one of the many 'freedom' rallies to decry restrictions that have been placed on the unvaxxed.

Despite their seeming ubiquity, all the experts I spoke to for this book (psychologists, social scientists, epidemiologists and others) told me that *true* anti-vaxxers – not the fearful, or the hesitant, or the time-poor, or the complacent, but the people who would stake their reputations and livelihoods on refusing to be vaccinated – are actually rare. By the end of summer 2021/22, upwards of 90 per cent of eligible Australians had been vaccinated against COVID-19, many of them having received three doses of one COVID vaccine, or of a mix of different COVID vaccines. People like my mother, who refuse to get vaccinated for ideological reasons and other deeply held beliefs, are a tiny – albeit incredibly vocal – minority here in Australia.

One problem, according to the experts I spoke to, is that these anti-vaxxers can persuade others, infecting the hesitant or anxious fence-sitters with the mistruths they cling to. Another is that they have become a lightning rod for activist groups with right-wing political ambitions and a desire to create chaos. The groups have coalesced into an angry mob whose separate origins and motivations have become hard to distinguish. Massive days- or weeks-long protests have taken place in Canada, the UK, France, Germany, Austria and New Zealand (to name a few), and, of course, here in Australia.

In February 2022, the Canberra Convoy, as it became known, drew an estimated 10,000 protesters to the nation's capital to protest vaccine mandates and other restrictions imposed during the pandemic. Emboldened by their sudden prominence on the world stage, militant anti-vaccine activists and their right-wing 'freedom fighter' allies have openly threatened violence on politicians and others. More protests are planned.

Online disinformation has also spilled over into personal attacks. In January, a Facebook user posted what was purported to be an eyewitness account falsely claiming that two girls at a Gold Coast medical clinic suffered violent convulsions and later died in the waiting room after receiving COVID-19 vaccinations. The post sparked panic and led to death threats against the doctor and clinic staff. The vicious reaction forced the clinic to pull out of the vaccine rollout to children aged five to eleven years, just three weeks after it began.

The COVID-19 vaccines – once billed as our ticket to freedom from lockdowns and masking and restrictions on visiting family and friends interstate and abroad – have instead turned out to be a spark that has fanned spot fires of discontent into nationwide protest movements. The daily barrage of headlines – about protests and court cases and unvaccinated sports stars – has continued unabated since vaccination against COVID-19 became freely available to most adults midway through 2021. Moral outrage flared on both sides, fuelling further coverage and commentary in the mainstream media.

When I spoke to Julie Leask, a social scientist who is the go-to expert on vaccine refusal, I asked her about the best way to combat anti-vaccine activists. Her advice: don't give them oxygen. 'Our perception of what others are doing affects what we think is a norm, and social norms affect vaccination,' she told me.

I've wrestled with this conundrum throughout my research and reporting for this book. By describing the reasons people have for refusing to be vaccinated, am I legitimising their position, lending weight to their arguments or, worse, drawing recruits to their cause? That is, of course, not my aim.

There are good reasons not to shy away from what is a complex and thorny issue. Vaccine coverage – though high – is far from uniform. For some, disadvantage and lack of access to vaccination services remain barriers. As a society – a wealthy one at that – we should all be concerned that this is the case. But we also need to take an unflinching look at why people who could access vaccines if they wanted to are instead refusing them, despite overwhelming support for vaccines from all corners of the scientific community and regulatory machinery.

In the first chapter, I try to make sense of who makes up the few per cent of people who haven't been vaccinated. Are they scared, complacent, stubbornly refusing vaccination? Or are they anti-vaxxers, actively promoting misinformation to recruit people into their fold?

The great unvaxxed are painted as selfish free-riders, relying on the goodwill and compliance of the rest of the community so that they can shirk their communal responsibilities. But what are their motivations for refusing vaccination? Chapter 2 examines the attitudes, personality traits and psychological roots of anti-vaccination sentiment.

The third chapter investigates the damage that is done with misinformation, which spreads rapidly through social media channels and private messaging apps. Rumours, inuendo and deliberate lies undermine public health programs and provoke anxiety in a public already unsettled by the uncertainties the pandemic has foisted upon them.

Some of the most successful creators and disseminators of anti-vax misinformation are scientists and medical practitioners. These bad actors use their professional clout and qualifications to bolster their credibility. Chapter 4 takes a look at some of the leading promulgators of anti-vaccination material and their outsized influence.

In chapter 5, I speak with people who have become ardent opposers of the coronavirus vaccines. Like my mother, they all have fingers in the complementary and alternative medicine or wellness industries. As these conversations reveal, shunning vaccination is a thread that runs deep in communities that also shun other forms of Western medicine.

Vaccine mandates are the spark that has ignited much of the outrage over COVID-19 vaccination. In chapter 6, I put vaccine mandates under the spotlight. Our response to people who are reluctant or unwilling to be vaccinated must be proportional to the threat that they pose. I ask whether vaccine mandates are the right tool to wield against this threat. It's a question that is particularly pertinent given the shifting landscape of the pandemic. Mandates enacted during the surge of the Delta variant in mid-2021 are being questioned – and in some instances abandoned – since the milder, more infectious and vaccine-dodging Omicron variant arrived on the scene.

In the US, vaccination rates – along with COVID-19 case numbers and deaths – can be overlaid onto maps of political affiliation. The Republican–Democrat right–left divide that is so stark in the US hasn't been replicated here, but anti-vaccine sentiment rubs up against libertarian and right-wing political ideologies as protests over vaccine mandates bring disparate groups together. This is the topic of chapter 7.

INTRODUCTION

Crystal-ball gazing is always a fraught affair, an invitation to be proven wrong. Nevertheless, the final chapter deals with how the pandemic – and vaccination – could play out from here, given what we know from the cresting and falling waves of infection that we've already seen.

The rift between my mother and me added to a sense that, in 2021, the pandemic took a turn from being a destructive and discombobulating force to being a truly divisive phenomenon. My hope is that close consideration of the unvaxxed pockets in our community – including their entanglement with free speech movements and questions of trust in government and the media – will help us to address this canary in the mine of broader societal discontent and disconnect. Out-of-hand dismissal of those who feel threatened by vaccine mandates, or who claim that their freedoms are being infringed, blinds us to the reasons that the anti-vaccine movement has become so prominent and ignores the serious consequences that might flow. A greater understanding of those at the fringe of our community will, I hope, illuminate ways that trust can be re-established and extreme outcomes – on a personal or societal level – can be avoided.

1.
UNVAXXED OR ANTI-VAX?

Talk to any vaccination expert in Australia about why some people remain unvaccinated – often stubbornly so – and they'll tell you to speak with Julie Leask. It's a recommendation I heard often in the early stages of writing this book. And in February 2022, I finally managed to set up a time to speak with Leask, a social scientist at the University of Sydney who has spent the past two decades trying to understand the unvaxxed.

Before our Zoom conversation really got going, Leask asked me about the book, what it was about, where I was coming from. I told her I wanted to understand vaccine hesitancy, why so many people refuse to be vaccinated, and why COVID-19 vaccinations had become such an incredible flashpoint in society. She listened as I explained my own personal interest in the topic, and blurted out a stream of disconnected ideas that I thought I could squeeze into the pages of the unwritten manuscript.

'Can I first challenge the ... sorry,' she interjected politely. 'I want to challenge you on the frame of the book.'

Hooo, boy, I thought. Have I already gone down the wrong path? 'Everybody's focused on hesitancy,' she said. 'It's the new buzzword for vaccination.'

Without a doubt, Leask said, there are people unsure about getting vaccinated, and unsure about the new COVID-19 vaccines in particular. They are concerned about the side effects, and worry that the vaccines are too new or have been too swiftly ushered through the regulatory checks and balances. Some are biding their time, waiting until they are reassured that the vaccines are safe enough, and that the alternative – rolling the dice with the coronavirus – is a bigger threat than their angst over vaccination. Indeed, many are unconvinced that a vaccine is even needed, perhaps secure in the belief that COVID-19 will not come for them – or, if it does, will leave them unharmed.

But hesitancy is frequently overplayed. And that makes Leask and other social scientists wince, especially if it's made out to be the only explanation for low vaccine uptake. In some contexts – where people need to work and look after children, or lack the ability to book or travel to appointments, for instance – vaccine hesitancy is only a minor player.

'Governments get off lightly if they can just blame what's going on in the heads of individuals, and not look at their failure to provide adequate services,' Leask said bluntly.

Framing the problem as one of hesitancy can be convenient. It paints the issue as one that lurks in the minds of the unvaxxed, not the problem of those of us who are vaccinated, not the government's problem. It takes the problem out of our collective hands, absolves us of responsibility and lays it in the laps of the few uninformed, misinformed or needlessly fearful.

The whole colourful spectrum of vaccine attitudes runs from the ardently pro-vaccination at one end, all the way to the steadfast refusers and anti-vax activists at the other. Leask dissects the unvaxxed into separate buckets. Several don't fit under the vaccine hesitancy banner at all. In one bucket are the 'can't haves' – people with specific medical conditions that mean they are unable to be vaccinated. In the context of COVID-19, the 'can't haves' also includes young children – at the time of writing – and, at various points during the first eight months of 2021, it included most adults who weren't elderly or otherwise prioritised for access when the rollout began in late February 2021.

Then there are the people who would get vaccinated if not for the insurmountable hurdles they face in making that happen. Parents with children to look after or migrant families unable to navigate the vaccine booking system fall into this bucket. So, too, do people in rural and remote communities who live far from their nearest health service.

In Victoria, the Pfizer vaccine was made available to people in their forties – my age group – in June 2021, amid a small but worrying outbreak of cases in the northern suburbs of Melbourne. I was keen to book my first shot. Booking an appointment close to home wasn't an option – GP clinics weren't yet part of the Pfizer rollout. So I would have to travel further afield, to a vaccination hub. That would have been fine, except that my daughter was home-schooling, and children were not allowed to attend the hubs. And so I waited, until – thankfully – schools reopened for a few brief weeks and I received both doses of the vaccine. I wasn't hesitant. I hadn't needed convincing that vaccination was in my and my community's best interests. And yet I waited, unable to access the vaccine when and where I wanted to.

For me, the hurdles were minor and temporary. But others are less fortunate. Across the country, vaccination rates for Indigenous Australians have lagged behind the average, in part because they have a harder time accessing vaccination services. Indigenous vaccine coverage trails non-Indigenous rates by 10 per cent or more in several states. In Western Australia and South Australia, the vaccination gap exceeds 20 per cent, according to data from February 2022.[1] Yet in August 2021, Indigenous affairs minister Ken Wyatt described the low uptake in Indigenous communities in the language of personal choice. 'Part of it is choice,' he told *The Guardian*. 'Some people have made choices because they've become fearful of adverse effects.'

Migrant communities with low levels of English and who lack the know-how to navigate the complex ecosystem of health services, as well as people without computers or smartphones to book appointments, also suffer disproportionately from an inability to access vaccination services. It is perhaps no surprise, then, that socially disadvantaged communities were hit hardest during the Omicron wave in Victoria. The poorest fifth of the community has the lowest vaccination rates and the highest death toll.

A year after the vaccine rollout began, more than 94 per cent of Australians aged sixteen and over had rolled up their sleeves for the first two doses of a coronavirus vaccine and nearly two-thirds had done so for a third 'booster' shot. Three-quarters of Australian twelve- to fifteen-year-olds were fully vaccinated, and just seven weeks into the rollout of the Pfizer vaccine to five- to eleven-year-olds, half had received their first dose. Figures are similar in New Zealand. Ninety-four per cent of Kiwis aged twelve and over are fully vaccinated, 72 per cent of adults have had a booster shot, and more than half of five- to eleven-year-olds have had their first dose.

The figures surpassed Leask's wildest expectations. 'I never dreamed it would get this high,' she told me, even knowing, as she does, that Australia's population is largely pro-vaccination. Coronavirus vaccine coverage in Australia and New Zealand is higher than most other nations. Higher than Canada and the US, higher than Japan, India and Brazil. Higher, of course than the dozens of poor nations across Africa, the Middle East and Asia that are desperate to secure doses to vaccinate their populations. Our closest neighbour, Papua New Guinea, has less than 4 per cent of its population vaccinated.

But getting where we are hasn't been smooth sailing. Since it began in Australia in late February 2021, the vaccine rollout has been marred by supply shortages, government missteps, and a confusing patchwork of policies that varied from state to state and month to month as vaccination opened to successively younger age blocks.

Over that time, blustery headwinds have shifted people in and out of vaccine hesitancy. There are those with concerns about safety – what Leask describes as 'medically hesitant'. There are people who are even more averse to vaccination but might still be convinced of its merit by, say, a trusted doctor. And then, in a bucket all their own, there are the trenchant objectors, who are completely against vaccination and are unlikely to be convinced otherwise.

In October 2020, three-quarters of Australians said they were willing to be vaccinated, according to data from the Taking the Pulse of the Nation survey that tracks how Australians feel about the coronavirus vaccines. But by February 2021, with the rollout about to start, that number had dropped to just two-thirds. Media reports comparing vaccine efficacy – information few would have known or been interested in for, say, the flu shot or the whooping cough vaccine – suddenly had people wondering about whether the vaccine about to be offered to them would even work.

For more than three months, vaccines were reserved for the elderly, frontline healthcare workers and other priority populations. By the start of June, federal government dithering meant that less than two-thirds of some of those groups – particularly aged and disability care residents and staff – had been vaccinated, even though care homes had repeatedly been the epicentre of COVID-19 deaths.

Meanwhile, GPs had been vaccinating people over fifty with the AstraZeneca shot since mid-March. But that rollout was also rocked by concerns about the safety of the vaccine, especially for women at the lower end of the age bracket. In April, the Australian Technical Advisory Group on Immunisation (ATAGI) – the body that advises how vaccines should be deployed – recommended against using the AstraZeneca vaccine in people younger than fifty, because of a rare blood-clotting disorder that authorities in Europe had linked to the shot. Australia's eagle-eyed media reported on every case of clotting that came to light, even some that later turned out to be unrelated to the vaccine. The proportion of people saying that they were unwilling or unsure about being vaccinated for COVID-19 peaked at 35 per cent of the population soon after.

ATAGI tightened its advice further in mid-June, making Pfizer the preferred shot for anyone under sixty years. By then, cases of the infectious Delta variant were blossoming in Sydney. With vaccines now available to forty- to forty-nine-year-olds, there was a sudden crush of demand for the Pfizer vaccine, outstripping the limited supplies that had arrived in the country.

At the end of the month, Prime Minister Scott Morrison threw petrol onto already simmering flames of uncertainty about the coronavirus vaccines. During a late-night press conference on 28 June, Morrison announced that the AstraZeneca vaccine would be available to all adults over eighteen who had consulted their doctors. GPs and public health bodies were blindsided, and a public war of words ensued. Some experts, including ATAGI, held firm on the advice to give younger people Pfizer rather than AstraZeneca, while others pointed to the successful rollout of AstraZeneca to young people in the UK as evidence that fears were exaggerated.

Many now became frustrated that people who could, if they wanted, get the AstraZeneca shot weren't lining up for it. Vaccine hesitancy was fingered as the culprit, and the hesitant as selfish and ignorant. But hesitancy was, for many, a reasonable response to the uncertainty being conveyed by politicians and the media, at a time when Australia's COVID-zero strategy meant the threat of death or serious illness from COVID-19 had touched few people directly. A simple cost–benefit assessment, where the risk from a disease outweighs the side effects of the vaccine designed to protect you, breaks down when the risk of disease is absent or intangible.

Once supply shortages began to ease in the second half of 2021, and with Australia's two largest cities in the grip of lockdown, governments started to pin an end to COVID-19 restrictions – for the vaccinated – to state-wide vaccination targets. Spurred on by the promise of a return to dining out, crowded bars, mask-less weddings, interstate travel, and funerals shared with loved ones, people dutifully lined up for their shots. Many who did so would have counted themselves among the hesitant just months or weeks earlier. But the added reassurance that came with family and friends being vaccinated, or the promise of a return to some version of 'normal', swayed them towards vaccination. The threat of being left out of the 'vaccinated economy' undoubtedly convinced others.

By October 2021, just 6.2 per cent of people remained firm in their opposition to the vaccine. That number has shifted little since, despite the widespread introduction of vaccine mandates, which require that workers in certain professions, ranging from nursing and dentistry to retail and hospitality, be vaccinated. Those who remain unvaxxed are assumed to be recalcitrant hold-outs – people who have selfishly decided to put their own ideologies above the health and functioning of our society.

We don't know how big this cohort of vaccine refusers would have been had history played out differently: had the AstraZeneca shot not been linked to blood clots, had more Pfizer shots been available sooner, had younger people been allowed access to vaccines earlier. Delays in vaccine rollouts can allow anxieties to fester and misinformation to percolate to the surface. As state and federal governments bickered over who should get what vaccine, and what vaccination target should trigger interstate borders to reopen, students to return to schools and groups to gather, trust in there being a single, science-guided 'truth' crumbled.

Before COVID-19, only a handful of Australians were in the bucket that Leask calls trenchant objectors – people who flat-out refuse to be vaccinated, or to let their children be vaccinated. Starting in 1996, when the Australian Immunisation Register began tracking childhood vaccinations, parents opposed to vaccines could register their conscientious objections, on personal, philosophical or religious grounds, after speaking with their doctor. Leask told me that this proviso was enough to drive vaccine refusal rates down well into the single digits. In 2013 – a year when more than 90 per cent of five-year-olds were fully vaccinated – Leask and her colleagues estimated that just 3.3 per cent of children, often concentrated in geographic pockets, were affected by vaccine-objecting parents. And only 1.8 per cent of those children were completely unvaxxed.[2]

That number had barely budged in more than a decade. Yet at the start of 2016, amid pressure and dedicated campaigning by the Murdoch press, the conscientious objection rule was binned with an introduction of the 'no jab, no pay' law. Whereas previously conscientious objectors had still qualified for family benefits from the government, the new law removed access to those benefits. State-based 'no jab, no play' laws restricting access to childcare for the unvaccinated were subsequently passed in New South Wales, Queensland, Victoria and Western Australia.

Childhood vaccination rates have crept slightly higher since those laws were introduced. Around 95 per cent of one-year-olds and a similar number of five-year-olds were fully vaccinated in September 2021. But it's not clear whether that's because there are fewer vaccine refusers, or whether access has been improved for those who were missing out.

Australia wasn't the only place where the noose was tightening around vaccine exemptions. In January 2015, an eruption of measles cases in the US was traced back to Disneyland in Anaheim, California. In all, 131 cases were scattered across California, and the virus was transported across borders into Arizona, Colorado, Nebraska, Oregon, Utah and Washington, as well as into Mexico and Canada. Two-thirds of the unvaccinated Californians who were infected in the outbreak had personal belief exemptions.

Later that year, California passed a law that banned non-medical exemptions. Vaccination rates in California rose after the law came into effect. But so too did medical exemptions. Vaccine refusal rates continued to soar in enclaves of like-minded parents, and in 2019 the US recorded more than 1200 measles cases across thirty-one states, the highest number of cases since the WHO declared the disease eradicated in the country in 2001. Alarmed, the international health agency listed vaccine hesitancy one of the top ten threats to global health in 2019.[3]

Anti-vax activists are a tiny slice of the already small minority of vaccine refusers. But they have become an increasingly vocal minority over recent years, in part because of their fight to stop changes to conscientious objector rules. When the COVID-19 pandemic hit, anti-vax activists were prepared with a well-thumbed playbook – downplaying the virus, exaggerating or outright lying about vaccine harms. And they had an established network on social media platforms ready to propagate those messages.

And this is where it becomes crucial to talk about vaccine hesitancy. Because those who are on the fence, deciding which way to go, can be nudged – like swing voters – towards vaccination, or away from it. Sometimes, those with the megaphone in your ear capture your attention first.

2.

MISTRUST AND THE ROOTS OF (DIS)BELIEF

At the end of January 2022, semi-trailers and freight haulers made their way across the frozen Canadian landscape, converging on the nation's capital of Ottawa. The 'Freedom Convoy' was sparked by a proposal that would make vaccination against COVID-19 mandatory for truck drivers entering Canada from the US. Not long after, protests emulating those in Ottawa kicked off in Canberra, Wellington and elsewhere. The demonstrations – part festival, part rabble-rousing cry for change – grew to be about more than just the vaccine mandates. But anti-vaccine sentiment was a fundamental trigger for the outrage.

If worried fence-sitters are at risk of becoming enthralled with anti-vax messages, I wanted to understand what attracts them, and what compels some to become ardent, active participants in a movement completely at odds with the scientific mainstream. I spoke to Matthew Hornsey, a social psychologist at the University of Queensland who studies why people reject scientific ideas that, to most, seem reasonable, or even self-evident: climate change is real, 5G mobile networks are safe, vaccines protect you.

Hornsey told me that most people, scientists included, don't have a good sense of why people reject science. They often conclude that people just don't understand it. Give them more information, in an easy-to-digest format, and they'll come around – or so the thinking goes. This is what's become known as the deficit model. If we could just heap on another spoonful of information, the message will get through.

Cartoonists and meme-creators play up this image of science deniers and vaccine refusers as ignoramuses lacking the requisite ability to discern accurate from inaccurate information. One cartoon by Tom Gauld, which was published in the popular science magazine *New Scientist*, shows the Devil introducing a newly arrived scientist to one of Hell's residents. The speech bubble reads: 'Welcome to science hell, Professor. This is Tony, he once saw something on the internet about your field of expertise and is going to spend eternity lecturing you on it.' In the era of COVID-19 vaccination, there have been numerous cartoon versions of a headstone in the cemetery. On it are etched the words, 'Here lies Jeff. He did his own research.'

The reality, says Hornsey, is that many anti-vaxxers genuinely do spend an inordinate amount of time poring over the latest scientific literature, reading vaccine studies or the lay explainers that follow on their heels. They frequently misconstrue the findings to fit their beliefs, or traipse down rabbit holes of blatantly inaccurate misinformation about cures no one else knows about. They alone have this valuable inside information. 'They're the ones doing the research,' says Hornsey, 'and we're sheep who just swallow what we're fed. When we imply that they're stupid or not doing their research, it's just exasperating for them.'

Hornsey told me that when faced with a decision, especially if there are shades of grey, he falls back on a rule of thumb. His is simple: trust the experts. It's a useful life-hack that most of us use to navigate the unfathomable complexity of modern life. What car do I purchase? Where do I send my kids to school? Should I rent this property?

In a global pandemic, Hornsey defers to public health authorities. 'I'll take the advice of the people who know best, and that's the scientists,' he said. When experts recommend a coronavirus vaccine that has been thoroughly assessed and has cleared all regulatory hurdles necessary, he'll take it.

We're often urged to use this kind of mental shorthand to judge sources of information, too. Want to avoid believing or – God forbid – sharing misinformation? Check that the source is reputable, we're told.

But at the heart of vaccine refusal – and the more virulent anti-vax activist movements – is a deep-seated sense of mistrust. Our willingness to trust a source or trust the recommendations of government and its institutions and advisers is indivisible from our trust in those sources. The lower the trust in authorities, the less likely someone is to take a risk – such as the risk of a vaccine side effect – even if the risk is tiny.

The irony, Hornsey said, is that when there's so much competing information – some real, some not, some trusted, some not – people fall back onto another mental shortcut. They rely not on the word of experts but on their own gut feelings and instinct, fuelled and coloured by fears, superstitions and personal bias. The mishmash of policies, or constant tweaks to public health recommendations, can further reinforce the idea that everything is a matter of opinion rather than scientific fact.

People are particularly susceptible to alternative sources of information when trust in traditional institutions has evaporated. In recent years, populist politicians from Donald Trump down have deliberately, and successfully, undermined the authority of mainstream media, academic experts and government agencies.

In other cases, the erosion of trust is of the government's own making. Over the past decade, Australia slid down Transparency International's Corruption Perceptions Index ranking, from seventh in the world in 2012 to eighteenth in 2021.[4] That was the largest drop of all thirty-eight members of the Organisation for Economic Co-operation and Development (OECD) bar Hungary, whose right-leaning government is actively pursuing policies to curtail democratic processes. In just a year, our scorecard suffered a 4-point hit, falling from 77 in 2020 to 73 in 2021 (where 100 is clean and 0 is highly corrupt). That's the equal largest drop over that time.

But you hardly need to look at international rankings to sense that there is seething mistrust in Australia. Since the start of the pandemic, political scandals have plagued governments of both persuasions. At the federal level, funding biases revealed in the 'Sports Rorts' scandal had barely subsided before the 'Car Park Rorts Affair' took hold. In 2021, Victoria's Labor government lost four ministers to a branch-stacking fiasco, and New South Wales lost its premier, Gladys Berejiklian, amid investigations into whether she breached public trust or encouraged corrupt behaviour. All the while, there has been growing exasperation that Australia has failed to put in place policies that adequately address the climate crisis. As the world is battered by bushfires and 'once-in-a-lifetime' storms and floods, fossil fuel projects are backed, not abandoned.

Scandals and government inaction all contribute to swirling suspicions that politicians and government institutions are unworthy of our trust. Or worse, they are secretive and harbour ulterior motives, aligning themselves with shady corporate interests over the interests of the people they serve.

Personal grievances, financial hardship – such as that brought on by the pandemic – or past run-ins with authorities can further heighten a person's sense of mistrust. People who lack trust – who have no simple 'trust the experts' rule of thumb – often find themselves in an almost impossible situation, where they take on the task of weighing risks and evaluating information themselves.

This is where peddlers of anti-vax misinformation can swoop in. People who are already anxious can be especially susceptible to groups that inflate vaccine harms and minimise the dangers of COVID-19. Indeed, we are all susceptible to this sort of narrative because it plays out in a cognitive quirk known as the omission bias. Simply put, we are more willing to accept the risk of doing nothing – in this case, not getting vaccinated – over the equal or lesser risk of doing something.

It's only in the last decade or so that researchers like Hornsey have probed the psychological underpinnings of vaccine refusal. In 2016, Hornsey and his colleagues surveyed more than 5000 people across twenty-four nations to identify the roots of anti-vaccination attitudes.[5]

One of the commonalities they discovered was disgust towards blood and needles. This makes sense. If you're afraid of needles, or you have an aversion to medical procedures and the places where they take place, you're more likely to come to the conclusion – rational or not – that vaccines do more harm than good. Taking a stance against vaccination could, in essence, be protective, a way of rationalising avoidance of a procedure that triggers fear and anxiety.

There are also certain personality traits that lead people to shun vaccines or join the anti-vax movement. One trait that popped out in Hornsey's data was what psychologists call 'reactance' and what others might uncharitably call pig-headedness. It's essentially an aversion to being told what to do, and those who measure high on the reactance scale are more likely to hold anti-vaccination sentiments.

What shocked Hornsey most, however, was that – more than any other factor measured – anti-vaccination attitudes were accompanied by a tendency towards conspiratorial beliefs. The relationship between the two was 'dramatic', he told me.

One of the hallmarks of conspiratorial thinking is distrust of authorities. So it's no surprise that anti-vax groups, much like people who promote COVID-19 conspiracy theories, attract people whose trust in government and mainstream media has already been shaken. The narrative that Big Pharma is colluding with government and medical regulators to hide data on vaccine side effects and wave through dangerous vaccines to line the pockets of executives is easy to believe for someone who already thinks those authorities are dishonest or crooked.

I spoke with Karen Douglas, a social psychologist at the University of Kent in the UK, to find out why people believe in conspiracies. She told me that pandemics and other unnerving world calamities are fertile ground for conspiracy theories to blossom. Fearful, anxious people suddenly don't understand the world around them. When people lose their jobs or are cut off from family and friends, they become even more susceptible to the lure of conspiracy theories, which offer people simple explanations for a seemingly inexplicable situation. 'Even people who might not be drawn to conspiracy theories normally might now start entertaining these ideas,' Douglas told me.

When the pandemic started in 2020, Douglas and her colleagues braced themselves. 'You start thinking, well, someone's going to come out and say that it's a hoax,' she said. 'And of course, that happened pretty much straightaway.' She also predicted that people would say the pandemic was planned, or blame specific countries for releasing the virus as a bio-weapon. Other theories – like the one about 5G mobile phone towers causing the pandemic – she didn't see coming.

Throughout history, pandemics have spawned conspiracy theories. When I spoke with psychologist and co-author of *The Conspiracy Theory Handbook*, Stephan Lewandowsky, he rattled off a long list of disease outbreaks where conspiracy theories have erupted. The Black Death in the Middle Ages was blamed on Jews poisoning water wells; HIV in the US was supposedly released by the Central Intelligence Agency to kill gay men; and in nineteenth-century Russia, doctors and nurses were chased down by a fearful public that thought them responsible for deaths during a cholera epidemic. 'Pandemics give rise to conspiracy theories, almost necessarily, whenever they occur,' Lewandowsky said.

Given the close relationship between vaccine refusal and conspiratorial worldviews, it's not surprising that vaccines are the object of several conspiracy theories. In 2015–16, the Zika virus swept through the Americas, causing a terrifying rise in cases of babies born with microcephaly – a condition marked by abnormally small heads and underdeveloped brains. Among the conspiracy theories that spread through the Americas, one suggested that pesticides were responsible, while another blamed genetically modified mosquitoes. Yet another popular conspiracy – propagated by anti-vax groups – was that expired measles-mumps-rubella (MMR) vaccines were to blame.

Fears about population control are so ubiquitous that conspiracy theories about vaccines causing infertility have emerged on numerous occasions. In Africa, rumours about the tetanus vaccine causing miscarriages in pregnant women started in the early 1990s in Kenya and continue to circulate to this day. In Nigeria, suspicions that the polio vaccine contained anti-fertility compounds led to a widespread boycott of the vaccine in the early 2000s. Fears that the human papillomavirus (HPV) vaccine causes women's ovaries to prematurely shut down lapped the Earth. And now, misinformation about the coronavirus vaccines causing infertility is pervasive in anti-vax messaging.

Although there are very real psychological needs that lead people to entertain or even seek out conspiracy theories, those theories rarely scratch the itch, Douglas told me. They might provide a seemingly plausible explanation, but they amp up anxieties and paranoia rather than providing solace. People find themselves in ever deepening mistrust, spiralling further and further down rabbit holes that confirm and reinforce their beliefs.

Because anti-vaccination sentiment and conspiratorial thinking involve a complex interplay between societal levels of trust and stability, as well as individual experiences and tendencies, tackling misinformation by correcting myths and debunking falsehoods can look like a band-aid solution applied to a festering wound. It can be an endless game of 'whack a mole' that ignores the underlying motivations and over-arching narratives that make myths stick.

Instead of debunking, Lewandowsky recommends what he calls 'inoculating' people. Others call it 'pre-bunking'. Just as a vaccine protects against a disease by training the body to recognise the contagion before it makes us sick, inoculating for contagious ideas trains people in advance to recognise where and when misinformation can flourish. An overlooked link in pre-bunking may be local doctors. One of the most important ways to prevent someone being recruited to the anti-vax movement is to make sure their experience with healthcare is a positive one, Julie Leask told me, and GPs are on the front lines of this experience.

Hornsey, meanwhile, argues that you need to strike at the attitudes and personal biases that underpin a person's belief in falsehoods. By way of illustration, Hornsey uses a tree metaphor. Above the surface are the visible leaves and branches, the superficial assertions that spill forth in conversations and online discussions. While it's tempting to scoff at these allegations and then send a link to an article online that helpfully debunks the claims, the fiercely held attitudes that lie under the surface – a distrust of pharmaceutical companies, for example – will likely remain.

Hornsey has applied this tree metaphor to discover the roots of climate change denial, and to think about ways of challenging those beliefs. In the case of climate change, people often reject the science because the personal cost of addressing the problem is too great. If someone doesn't like the prospect of giving up their gas-guzzling car or their intercontinental flights, they might reject the science that suggests they downsize their car or fly less often. Others might reject climate science for ideological reasons. Perhaps they are opposed to so-called 'big government' interventions that would raise the costs for polluting businesses and curb free enterprise.

Appeals to these root sensibilities can sway peoples' opinions, Hornsey says. For example, laying out the economic arguments for reducing harmful emissions or demonstrating that there are free-market–friendly ways of slowing global warming can make people more likely to embrace the science of climate change rather than dismiss it out of hand.

But whereas climate change has only a few large taproots lying under the surface, the subterranean foundations of vaccine rejection resemble a Medusa-like tangle of intertwined motivations. 'It defies a simple prescription,' Hornsey told me.

In this sense, vaccine rejection is a quintessential 'wicked problem', at once hard to grasp and defying a simple one-size-fits-all solution. Tailored outreach efforts that topple any and all access barriers must be paired with deft communication campaigns to arm people against misinformation. But that alone won't be enough. Given the right circumstances – as the pandemic has proven – doubts can be fanned into raging fires of suspicion. And if the government, mainstream media, and even our employers, families and friends dismiss us or lose our trust, we can be left searching for answers in the darker corners of our online worlds.

3.
NETWORKS OF HARM

The website for Australia-based Parents With Questions is slick and professional. Scrawled across the front page in all-caps chalkboard-style lettering is their opening gambit: 'We love our kids. And as parents we have a few serious questions about COVID-19 vaccinations. How about you?' Scroll further down and a neat grid of embedded videos pops up to greet you – they are parents, and they have questions, they each tell you.

Rollout of the Pfizer vaccine for kids aged twelve and above started in the US, Italy and elsewhere in May 2021. Since then, children have become the new frontier in the battle against COVID-19 vaccination. On the 'About' page of the Parents With Questions website is a section titled 'Where it all began', which describes the day 'PWQ' was born. Founder and father of three Adam Gibson 'sat around a campfire' with Jon Farriss, of INXS fame, and another neighbour, Charlie Arnott, to do something about the impending rollout of COVID-19 vaccines to children aged five to eleven years.

When I spoke to Gibson in February 2022, he launched into this campfire origin story. How he and his mates felt 'very concerned', he said, and 'also a bit powerless'. But a few minutes into the conversation, he conceded there was another backstory to PWQ's beginnings. 'This is what actually prompted it, I'll give you the full story,' he said.

Before that fireside discussion, Gibson – a farmer and Byron Bay–based sustainable food business consultant – called the office of Justine Elliot, his local Labor MP. He was concerned about the adverse reactions that the Therapeutic Goods Administration (TGA) was reporting on its website, he told the person who answered his call. Over 400 deaths were reported to have occurred within two weeks of vaccination, but all bar seven were deemed to be unrelated to the vaccine. 'How could that be?' he wondered. The staffer suggested Gibson put his concerns in writing, which he did and emailed Elliot's office on 13 August 2021. Why were the seven deaths not being reported along with COVID-19 cases, he asked, and who has determined that the other deaths were not related to the vaccines?

He received no response, so he called Elliot's office again. The staffer who answered this time wasn't as cordial as the first. 'He got really heated,' Gibson told me. The staffer accused Gibson of relying on Trump conspiracy sites, and ended the conversation yelling at Gibson to, 'Go get vaccinated and get a fucking life.' A spokesperson for Elliot's office denies such a call took place.

Incensed, Gibson took this as a clear indication that something sinister was afoot. Public officials could not be trusted to be transparent and divulge the information necessary for people to make an informed decision about vaccination. More than a lack of transparency, there was likely a cover-up happening.

The call lit a flare for Gibson. That's when the fireside chat happened and soon after, he and nine other like-minded friends banded together, amassing between them a 'fighting fund' of more than $100,000. Their initial goal was to mount a legal case against the politicians they said were failing to represent their constituents by withholding information about adverse events resulting from vaccination. A 'Nuremberg 2.0' trial is how he referred to the legal case in a Facebook livestream broadcast with the Great Australian Party senate candidate Jason Miles on 1 December 2021. Gibson isn't the first to liken government actions during the pandemic to those of the Nazis.

No lawyer would take the case. The group were also rebuffed from purchasing billboard ads across the nation. Failing that, they turned to online marketing, and PWQ was launched, both as a website and as an active presence on social media. PWQ joined an already thriving ecosystem of online anti-vax messaging.

The modern anti-vax movement was launched in the late 1990s after the medical journal *The Lancet* published a now-infamous study by British physician-turned-activist Andrew Wakefield connecting the MMR vaccine to autism. The study was tiny, reporting on just twelve children whose developmental disorders were potentially linked to the vaccine. The paper couldn't say for sure that the vaccine caused the children's conditions, but at a press conference Wakefield's conclusions were clear. 'I can't support the continued use of these three vaccines given in combination until this issue has been resolved,' he said.

Since then, the study has been thoroughly debunked, and millions of dollars have been spent on additional studies that comprehensively show no link between the MMR vaccine and autism exists. In 2004, British journalist Brian Deer revealed that some of the parents of the children in Wakefield's paper were recruited by a lawyer preparing to launch a class action against the MMR vaccine manufacturer. Wakefield was personally paid more than £400,000 to help build the case, and stood to make even more money as the patent holder of a single measles vaccine that would rival the combination MMR shot. The *Lancet* paper was fully retracted in 2010, and Wakefield was struck off the UK medical register three months later.

By then, the damage was done. Wakefield's paper was published at the dawn of the internet era, and news of its false claims spread unimpeded around the world. Vaccination rates fell sharply in the UK, and in 2019, the country lost its measles-free status. Outbreaks in the US – declared free of measles in 2001 – became more common. And the

MMR autism rumours continue unabated, the misinformation unable to be scrubbed from the internet and the tentacles of its social media platforms.

In Australia, the leading anti-vax activist group is the Australian Vaccination-risks Network. The group was founded in 1994 as the Vaccination Awareness Network by American-born Meryl Dorey, who subsequently changed the name to the Australian Vaccination Network. The group was forced to change its name again after the New South Wales Office of Fair Trading deemed the name to be 'misleading and a detriment to the community' in 2012. It adopted the name Australian Vaccination-sceptics Network in 2014, and then settled on Australian Vaccination-risks Network in 2018.

Despite the convoluted history of the group's name, its mission, since its inception, has been to oppose vaccines and vaccine mandates at every turn. Since the beginning of the pandemic, the group has trotted out the usual COVID-19 conspiracies and vaccine misinformation – that the pandemic was intentionally released (#plandemic), that the virus is no worse than the flu (#scamdemic), and the vaccines have been rushed to market, are experimental, don't work, and could put you at risk of sudden death.

With COVID-19, groups like the Australian Vaccination-risks Network, forged to denounce childhood vaccinations, have been joined by fledgling political parties, not-for-profit charities, discussion forums and ragtag groups of grassroots activists. The interconnected groups form an echo chamber, disseminating emotion-laden messages, usually from just a small coterie of prolific anti-vax influencers, to obliterate public support for COVID-19 vaccinations.

Between January 2020 and March 2021, membership nearly tripled for thirteen public Facebook groups based in Australia that were spreading anti-vax messages, according to the charity Reset Australia, which tracks online misinformation.[6] Surges in membership numbers and engagement – likes, shares and comments, for instance – coincided with lockdowns in 2020.

PWQ started with the modest ambition of reaching five million people through Facebook and Instagram in the six weeks leading up to Christmas 2021. They smashed that goal, according to Gibson, instead reaching 23.9 million people. At the end of February 2022, the PWQ website claimed to have 15,000 subscribers, and its Telegram account had amassed more than 10,000 subscribers, more than on its Facebook or Instagram pages, which are relaunched as 2.0, 3.0, 4.0 versions each time Facebook or Instagram ban them.

Anti-vax activism is now a predominantly online endeavour. Mathew Marques, a social psychologist at La Trobe University, recalls that when he was a teen in the 1990s, a co-worker at his part-time supermarket job handed him a relic of the time – a zine filled with offbeat information about UFOs and free energy conspiracy theories. 'That was how you got your information,' he said. Finding information in bookstores or via the clunky pre-Google internet would have prevented all but the most dedicated from accessing anti-vax information.

Social media changed all of that, said Marques, who studies how people form their views on contentious scientific topics – from climate change and genetically modified foods to vaccination.

One reason social media platforms are such an effective – and harmful – vehicle for activists is that they give people the illusion of numbers. Anti-vax communities used to occur in geographical clusters. But on social media, fringe beliefs can amass large online communities. And because the desire to belong to a group and follow societal norms is ingrained in our evolutionary make-up, members of the group tend to adopt the behaviours being promoted. If everyone you encounter online shuns vaccination, it's likely you will be swayed to as well. And once you're hooked into an anti-vax community, platform algorithms reinforce your connection to similar groups. While I was writing this book, a notification popped up on Facebook. 'Based on Pages that you've interacted with, you might like Jobs without Jabs Victoria,' it said, directing me to a private group with close to 4000 members.

In August 2021, *CBS Mornings* anchor Gayle King asked Facebook CEO Mark Zuckerberg how many people on Facebook had viewed and shared posts containing misinformation about COVID-19 vaccines. He deflected the question. 'A lot of the stuff that's actually the hardest for us to really address is not what I would call "misinformation" but instead another category that I would call "hesitancy",' he told King. Hesitant or not, many Facebook users are not getting vaccinated. A July 2021 study by researchers at Northwestern University found that the vaccination rate for Americans who used Facebook as their only source of COVID-19 information was a whopping 40 per cent lower than for those who found their information elsewhere.[7]

The PWQ mission is, ostensibly, to encourage parents to ask their own questions and make up their own minds about vaccinating their kids against COVID-19. Leask wasn't familiar with the PWQ site when we spoke, but she told me that this kind of sophisticated 'wolf in sheep's clothing' approach is becoming more common. Smouldering doubts are fanned with innocent-sounding – yet impossible to answer – questions and anodyne advice. 'Listen to that voice inside us that's whispering, "What if they're wrong?"' implores the PWQ website. 'Say "no" until we are 100% sure.'

When pressed, Gibson concedes that the site discourages vaccination of children, and that his reservations about vaccines pre-date the rollout to children. Gibson himself is unvaccinated against COVID-19. When one of his daughters was a toddler, he and his wife – 'on medical advice' – decided to delay their daughter's vaccinations. For two years, while she was excluded from childcare, Gibson became a stay-at-home father.

The PWQ brand limits its purview to COVID-19 vaccines for children, but the group has sponsored a misconstrued report on COVID-19 vaccine effectiveness across age groups by another anti-vax group, People for Safe Vaccines. Whatever the target, those behind PWQ draw on a familiar anti-vax playbook: vaccines are far more dangerous than we're led to believe, and the risks of COVID-19 are exaggerated; it's taking a sledgehammer to crack a nut. 'All risk, no reward,' as Gibson puts it.

Indeed, many of the 'scamdemic' conspiracies that cropped up early in the pandemic were propagated by anti-vax activist groups already active. Downplaying the severity of COVID-19, or claiming outright that the pandemic was an elaborate hoax, helped to undermine the vaccines well ahead of their rollout.

Gibson's job of sowing doubt in the minds of parents has been made easier by the emergence of a rare side effect of the mRNA-based vaccines. Males under thirty – and females to a lesser extent – can develop inflammation of the heart muscle (myocarditis) or surrounding tissue (pericarditis) in the days following vaccination. The condition is rare enough that the clinical trials didn't pick it up. And experts are quick to point out that the condition is mild, it is treatable, and you're more likely to get it from COVID-19 than you are from the vaccine.

It's a fear that anti-vax groups play on. A COVID-19 factsheet, downloadable from the PWQ website, warns parents that 'adverse effects from these vaccines may affect young people for life, leading to myocarditis, autoimmunity problems, cancers, and potentially death'.

But the factsheet has some reassuring news for parents about COVID-19. 'The disease in children is extremely mild and may only be a runny nose, cough or many have tummy upset as the lymph glands in their tummies become swollen,' it reads. 'The recovery rate is 99.99%', it continues, 'and healthy children don't seem to have ongoing health issues'. The factsheet also makes the false claims that 'COVID-19 vaccines available in Australia are experimental and still under research', and that 'there is very little data to demonstrate that children are spreaders of the virus'.

George Christensen, the conservative Queensland Liberal National Party politician, used similar language when talking to Meryl Dorey, founder of the Australian Vaccination-risks Network, in February 2022. 'In my world, you don't go and inject a whole cohort of children for something that, in its deadly phase, caused an outbreak of runny noses,' he said, referring to data from the Delta wave in mid-2021. 'Kids get runny noses all the time. I don't need to vaccinate my kid for a runny nose.'

I asked paediatrician and vaccine researcher Jim Buttery from the Murdoch Children's Research Institute whether Gibson – and others – had a point about there being a lack of transparency. The US Centers for Disease Control and Prevention attracted all the wrong sorts of attention in February 2022 when a *New York Times* article revealed that the agency had held onto large swathes of COVID-related data – from wastewater analyses to the effectiveness of booster shots in certain age groups.[8] If health agencies were more forthcoming with data, I asked, would that assuage concerns, or at least remove a cudgel from the hands of the anti-vax groups who wield it?

Buttery – a member of the TGA's Advisory Committee on Vaccines – doesn't think so. 'Surveillance is dirty data,' he told me, and it takes time to find the signal of vaccine-caused symptoms and side effects in the noise of symptoms that merely occur post-vaccination by chance. The anti-vax lobby also has a long history of misinterpreting this data, precisely because it presents as a frightening list of adverse events. That is what Craig Kelly, former Liberal Party MP and now United Australia Party leader, was counting on when he sent unsolicited text messages in September 2021 directing people to information taken from the TGA's Database of Adverse Event Notifications. The information is not incorrect, but it provides no context about the seriousness of the illnesses reported, nor whether they are in any way related to the vaccine.

What you won't find on the PWQ factsheet is any mention of a rare but sometimes deadly condition called multisystem inflammatory syndrome in children (MIS-C) that is estimated to affect as many as 1 in 3000 children and often hits perfectly healthy kids two to six weeks after a mild bout of COVID-19. You also won't find any mention of children developing long COVID, the debilitating post-viral condition that can linger for weeks or months following infection. Vaccines protect against both of these COVID-related conditions but don't fit the PWQ narrative.

Other attempts to sway opinion and incite outrage are far more blatant. 'Everyone, I lost my son Lachlan last Wednesday to the vaccine. He was 7 yrs old', reads an emotional post that appeared on Facebook soon after primary school–aged children started rolling up their sleeves to get a first dose of the Pfizer vaccine in January 2022. 'The government has ruined my family, they have taken away our only son, we put out trust in the government to keep us safe and they killed my boy!!!'

The heart-wrenching story that unleashed panic on social media was quickly revealed to be a hoax. There was no distraught father, no grief-stricken, sedated mother, no seven-year-old boy in a coffin because of a vaccine-induced heart attack. The profile picture of 'Steve Leary' – the father in the tall tale – had been filched from an actual Steve Leary, the mayor of Winter Park, part of the metropolitan sprawl of Orlando, Florida.

Fake stories like this stick, tugging at our emotions and fertilising small seeds of doubt in our minds. Once seen, they are hard to unsee. And once set free on social media, they spread faster and wider than information that later exposes their fakery.

The fall-out from vaccine panic can be devastating. In 2010, Japan started vaccinating teenage girls with the human papillomavirus (HPV) vaccine to prevent cervical cancers caused by strains of the virus, and within three years, about 70 per cent of girls were getting the shot. But rumours and media reports of teenagers fainting after receiving the vaccine spooked the Japanese government, which stopped proactively recommending the vaccine.

The consequences of the panic were twofold. The fainting episodes were most likely a case of mass psychogenic illness, a psychological reaction that can spread from person to person, such as when schoolgirls watch each other getting and then reacting to the vaccine. YouTube clips and reports of fainting can further prime people for a negative reaction. A similar bout of post-jab reactions occurred in an Iranian class administered with tetanus shots, and in twenty-three Taiwanese schools after the flu shot.

HPV vaccine rumours also spread through Colombia and Denmark, but it was only in Japan that the recommendation to vaccinate was suspended. The vaccination rate cratered to less than 1 per cent. At the end of 2021, researchers estimated that a single year of the suspension – which has now gone on for eight and a half years – could translate into an additional 3700 cases of cervical cancer and 900 deaths from the disease.[9] The Japanese government finally corrected course in November 2021, advising local governments to resume HPV vaccination.

Groups like PWQ and the Australian Vaccination-risks Network prefer not to be tarred with the anti-vax label. They instead claim to encourage curiosity, and to level a playing field distorted by censorship of vaccination information. They argue that their approach fosters informed vaccination choice, yet distort the information they share. They lean on personal anecdotes of unsubstantiated vaccine injuries, and as their membership and monetary support blooms, their sophistication ripens along with it. The most successful anti-vax campaigners fund slick documentaries that are professionally produced and distributed. As we shall see, those who rise to the top have an outsized influence in online spaces, with smaller groups acting as their diligent local mouthpieces.

4.
BAD ACTORS

I first heard of Robert Malone in June 2021, when his wife, Jill, sent an email to me – and who knows how many other journalists – to 'set the record straight'. Her husband of forty-two years, she wrote, was wrongly being written out of history as the inventor of mRNA vaccination. 'This was and is Robert's work, his passion,' she went on to say. 'He is thrilled that all these technologies are working.'

The Pfizer and Moderna vaccines both use mRNA technology, the first in history to do so. They work by injecting a protein's genetic instructions – the mRNA – into the body, rather than the more traditional approach of injecting the protein itself. The effect is the same. The body's immune system detects the protein – whether it's made in-house by the body or injected – and in the process is trained to recognise and vanquish the virus carrying that protein.

Despite the sameness for the body, mRNA vaccines mark a technological revolution that is widely touted as deserving of a Nobel Prize for its inventors.

But according to Jill's email, the mainstream media was giving that credit to others – the scientists at Moderna and BioNTech whose work finally produced the now-famous vaccines – even though Malone's own 'seminal work' in the field, wrote Jill, is what 'spawned the mRNA vaccination technologies now saving the world from COVID-19'. It is true that Malone's experiments as a graduate student at the Salk Institute for Biological Studies in La Jolla, California, in the 1980s and early 1990s were, at the very least, crucial stepping stones along the path to mRNA vaccine discovery. But how Malone's contribution measures up against the work of scientists who came before and after is one that is no doubt being debated by prize committees in Sweden and elsewhere.

In the months since that email, Malone has risen in acclaim, not for championing the vaccines his lab experiments contributed to, but for cutting them down every chance he gets. In January 2022, Malone's popularity reached its zenith after he appeared on one of America's most popular podcast shows, *The Joe Rogan Experience*. When the episode was released on 31 December 2021, it went out to more than eleven million listeners.

Health experts were appalled. The podcast contained a litany of falsehoods and misleading statements about the mRNA vaccines. Between insinuating that US President

Joe Biden is unvaccinated, that elite athletes were dropping dead after being vaccinated and that the vaccines are experimental, Malone leaned on his well-worn claims that the mRNA vaccines have been rushed through approvals far too swiftly, without any consideration for long-term side effects that might appear. He and others make this claim about a lack of long-term data because it's hard to dispute – the vaccines are new, after all. But vaccines don't produce longer-term side effects. Any reactions, if they occur, do so in the minutes, days or at most weeks following vaccination.

Hundreds of doctors, nurses, scientists and educators wrote an open letter to Spotify, which hosts *The Joe Rogan Experience*, urging the streaming platform to 'take action against the mass-misinformation events' on its service. Musicians Neil Young and Joni Mitchell removed their music from Spotify, along with podcasters Roxanne Gay and Mary Trump, Donald Trump's niece. YouTube has removed the episode that users uploaded to the site, but Spotify refused to bow to pressure and the whole three-hour episode remains on the platform.

Malone's meteoric rise in anti-vax circles has been aided in no small part by his qualifications. He's a scientist. He didn't just work on – he literally *invented*, according to him – the technology he is now tearing down. He's the best kind of insider the anti-vax lobby could lay their hands on. And Malone has been more than obliging to lend his credentials to the cause.

The ploy works. I spoke to Mel, a woman who left her hometown and a job with a vaccine mandate to make a documentary film about the untold stories of people injured by coronavirus vaccines. She said to me, 'Who am I to argue with Dr Malone who has nine patents for mRNA technology? He's saying don't get these jabs. I'm not going to argue with him.'

Medical experts and scientists who lend their voices to the anti-vaccination lobby are invariably painted as brave rank-breakers, people who have uncovered a truth that is being kept from the public by corrupt authorities. And Malone is just one among a cast of celebrity scientists and physicians who anti-vax activists use to promote their position.

The tactic was honed long before COVID-19 came along. When Andrew Wakefield launched his career as a vaccine naysayer, he had a colossal ace up his sleeve – he was a qualified doctor, and a scientific researcher to boot. As much as the anti-vaccination activists shun the mainstream and fob off expert advice from health authorities, they frequently lean on the veneer of credibility that a 'qualified expert' can provide.

In Australia, vaccinologist Nikolai Petrovsky at Flinders University in Adelaide has fashioned himself into a home-grown counterpart to Malone. Petrovsky – whose company, Vaxine, has developed a protein-based vaccine called COVAX-19 – has disparaged mRNA vaccines as 'gene therapies' rather than vaccines, and as 'experimental', and has said that the vaccines approved so far lack long-term safety data. The claims are inaccurate and misleading but have gained Petrovsky a following among Australia's unvaxxed. Petrovsky is currently on long service leave from his position at Flinders University because he has refused to be vaccinated with an approved vaccine, having already received shots of his company's COVAX-19. Petrovsky did not respond for comment.

One thing attracting some to Petrovsky's vaccine – though it is also lacking in long-term safety data and is as yet unproven in humans – is that Petrovsky doesn't represent the interests of Big Pharma. He has painted himself as the David to Big Pharma's Goliath, a struggling local researcher forced to crowdfund his work while the government shovels billions into the pockets of Pfizer and AstraZeneca.

Non-expert celebrities can also affect vaccine acceptance because of the sheer size of their audience. In September 2021, rapper Nicki Minaj tweeted a message of warning to her twenty-four million followers. 'My cousin in Trinidad won't get the vaccine cuz his friend got it and became impotent,' she tweeted. 'His testicles became swollen. His friend was weeks away from getting married, now the girl called off the wedding.' She ended the tweet with her sage advice: 'So just pray on it & make sure you're comfortable with ur decision, not bullied.' The tweet has been liked nearly 150,000 times and retweeted without comment close to 25,000 times.

On 17 January 2022, Malone shared his views on an episode of George Christensen's *Conservative One* podcast.

The episode, provocatively titled 'Do not vax your children! – with Dr Robert Malone', drew instant rebukes from across the political spectrum. Prime Minister Scott Morrison urged parents to ignore Christensen's 'dangerous messages', but he was heavily criticised for failing to expel Christensen from the party room and pull into line other MPs in his party who were sowing doubt and misinformation about coronavirus vaccines.

By the end of the month, Malone was presenting his views alongside anti-vax royalty – Robert F. Kennedy Jr – at the 23 January 'Defeat the Mandates' rally in Washington, DC. Aside from being part of the country's most famous political family, RFK Jr, as he is known, is one of the best known anti-vaxxers globally. Since the 1980s, he has built a reputation as a formidable and talented environmental lawyer. But his name is now synonymous with the anti-vax movement. In 2011 he founded Children's Health Defense – formerly the World Mercury Project – which is one of the most prolific dispensers of anti-vaccine misinformation online. During the COVID-19 pandemic, his popularity surged even higher. Well before COVID-19 vaccinations were available to the general public, RFK Jr spread falsehoods and doubt about everything from facemasks and the severity of COVID-19 to the nefarious influence of Bill Gates on global vaccine policy.

Vaccine scepticism in the US also got a boost from Donald Trump's rise to the White House, according to social psychologist Matthew Hornsey. In the decade before he became president in 2017, Trump espoused anti-vaccination views, talking and tweeting about how vaccines cause autism. Although he largely sidestepped the topic once in office, his views sowed a seed of doubt in the minds of his supporters.

Several unvaxxed people I spoke to for this book told me that they were disappointed with Trump. Not because of his repeated lies while in office, or his role in instigating the storming of the US Capitol building on 6 January 2021, or the numerous other acts and utterances that outraged many people during his presidency. Instead, they are disappointed that Trump missed a grand opportunity. He failed to follow through on his 2016 promise to have RFK Jr – who sits at the pinnacle of anti-vax networks – to chair a commission on vaccines once he was elected.

In March 2021, the UK-based not-for-profit Center for Countering Digital Hate (CCDH) listed RFK Jr as number two – behind osteopath and natural health news site entrepreneur Joseph Mercola – on its 'Disinformation Dozen', a list of the most prolific anti-vax super-spreaders on social media at the time.[10] Between them, these twelve celebrities and their organisations generated 65 per cent of the anti-vaccination content shared on Facebook and Twitter over a six-week period from the beginning of February 2021. Over that time, CCDH estimated that there were more than sixty-two million followers of anti-vaccine accounts on Facebook, Instagram and Twitter.

The prominence on social media of a handful of anti-vax voices is why de-platforming – yanking them from the social media platforms they operate on – can limit their sphere of influence. Malone was removed from Twitter the day before his sit-down with Joe Rogan, losing him more than half a million followers. But other platforms are ready and waiting to take the place of Facebook, Twitter and YouTube.

Since Malone was ousted from Twitter, he has turned to platforms I'd never heard of before writing this book. They include the Twitter alternative GETTR, where he already has close to 360,000 followers, gab (149,000 followers) and Telegram (11,000 subscribers). He also communicates with followers via the subscription newsletter service Substack. On 27 January 2022, CCDH estimated that Substack generates at least US$2.5 million annually – and as much as US$12.5 million – from the combined income of the top five anti-vax newsletters it hosts.[11] Newsletters by Joseph Mercola and Robert Malone are among those.

There is also money to be made from book deals and sales. Malone's book, *Lies My Gov't Told Me and the Better Future Coming*, is set to be published in June 2022. And RFK Jr's *The Real Anthony Fauci: Bill Gates, Big Pharma, and the Global War on Democracy and Public Health* has already made its way to as high as number five on the *New York Times* bestseller list.

Social media platforms are under constant pressure to root out vaccine misinformation and the people who spread it. In August 2021, Facebook CEO Mark Zuckerberg said that the platform had removed eighteen million posts containing misinformation about vaccines. Yet some big names, including RFK Jr and his Children's Health Defense, remain on the site.

Of course, de-platforming plays right into the narrative that anti-vaxxers are selling: that they are being censored so that the inconvenient truth doesn't come out. But in Stephan Lewandowsky's eyes, it's a strategy that works. Their audience is reduced and they are no longer able to convert the fence-sitters, the sceptical and hesitant people who might fall either way given the right nudge.

When Malone appeared on *The Joe Rogan Experience* he also blew new life into the 'mass psychosis' nonsense that I'd first heard about from my mother five months earlier. In anti-vax circles – and more so in conspiracy theory communities – people who get vaccinated or go along with government recommendations are mocked as 'sheeple', hapless dupes who blindly follow propaganda dutifully broadcast by an equally credulous – or complicit – mainstream media. 'Mass psychosis' – or 'mass formation psychosis' as Malone called it – is a more extreme incarnation of this idea, where entire populations fall prey to propaganda messages seemingly so powerful that they hold people in their thrall, leading them to march off to vaccination clinics against their will.

The idea has echoes of terms like 'mob mentality' and 'group mind'. But it's essentially bunk, according to social psychologist Stephen Reicher from the University of St Andrews in Scotland, who has been studying crowd psychology for more than four decades. After Malone floated the idea on Rogan's show, Reicher was blunt in his assessment of the motives behind such ideas. 'Telling people who disagree with you that they are deluded and in a state of psychosis is essentially a device to silence them and a form of disrespect,' he told the AP news agency.

Talk of mass psychosis breeds divisions. People who are unsure about whether the vaccines recommended to them are safe or necessary are right to get their hackles up when their concerns are dismissed as those of lunatics and imbeciles. By the same token, Malone's taunt dismisses anyone who follows mainstream media as moronic, unable to think for themselves. Disparaging each other in this way divides the world into 'them' and 'us' camps, fracturing personal relationships and deepening mistrust.

Malone and his ilk are frighteningly successful in promoting their message. Their charisma and expertise convince many. Their words become truth, arming the unvaxxed with a weapon against those who question their decision. If the doctor says the vaccines are bad, who am I to say otherwise? And who are you?

5.
AN ATTEMPT TO SWINDLE NATURE

On a grey and muggy morning in February 2022, I drove south along Beach Road, winding past bayside suburbs of southeast Melbourne, the ocean a dark steely blue to my right. At a beachside park I met up with three women, all close to retirement age by my estimation, and all unvaxxed.

Over the next couple of hours, Judy, Maureen and Noela told me their stories. Each was unique, shaping their concerns into distinct configurations. But there were common threads – their lives spent in caring professions, their disillusionment with mainstream medicine, and their deep suspicions about the coronavirus vaccines and the forces that have made them mandatory. They have become pariahs among family and friends, and have found solace in the communities of unvaccinated people they have found online and at political rallies.

Noela originally trained as a nurse and midwife. For years, she travelled town to town around Victoria, administering tuberculosis shots to children. In February 2021, she completed her immunisation provider certification, readying herself to administer the new Pfizer vaccine as the rollout ramped up. But she never ending up doing that. After completing the course she took a break, during which she became a grandmother and prepared for ankle surgery.

That's when she started seeing red flags. First were the blood clots from the AstraZeneca vaccine. In her own experience as a nurse, she'd only ever witnessed one person have a serious reaction to a vaccine – in that case a potent allergic reaction, or anaphylaxis. But the media was constantly reporting on this new side effect, and countries were scrambling to review the vaccine's rollout. With ankle surgery looming, anything that could raise Noela's risk of getting a post-operative blood clot seemed incredibly dangerous.

While she waited for the Pfizer vaccine to be available in her age group – and with her fears already piqued – she saw another red flag: the changing vaccination schedule. When the Pfizer vaccine was approved, the two shots were recommended to be taken three weeks apart. With demand for the vaccine far outstripping supply in mid-2021, authorities in Victoria changed the schedule, recommending at the beginning of August that the two doses be given six weeks apart. There were also changes to the AstraZeneca schedule. New South Wales slashed the wait between first and second doses from twelve weeks to just four, and in Victoria the wait was cut to six weeks.

The rationale for these changes was that it was better to have most people partially vaccinated than only a few fully vaccinated. It was a strategy that the UK had employed earlier in 2021, and it had worked to bring rates of infection, hospitalisation and death down. But in Noela's eyes, the shifting recommendations were suspicious. Never in her time as a nurse had she seen a vaccination schedule change like this.

Then came another red flag with the introduction of Moderna into the mix. People could choose which vaccine to get, which seemed ridiculous to Noela. How could vaccines be interchangeable like that? Her dread had now grown to encompass all COVID-19 vaccines available in Australia.

A final, damning red flag was the vaccine side effects. Noela told me that she knows eight people who have had a COVID-19 vaccine and reacted to it. One is her son-in-law, who got pericarditis – a known and treatable side effect of the mRNA-based shots – after his first dose. There's no way for me to know how serious any of these side effects were, but they clearly spooked Noela.

While these red flags were appearing, Noela had two thoughts churning in her mind. The first was the knowledge that her son and his fiancée had caught, and survived, COVID-19 during England's first wave in early 2020. Noela likened what her son had to a mild case of 'man flu'. The second was that there was no one in Australia who she knew personally that had caught the virus. So, why should a healthy woman like her get vaccinated?

Red flags are all Noela sees now. Her nursing career is all but over. Her registration has lapsed, and she has no plans to return to the job, because she would need to be vaccinated to do so. She has paid a high price in friendships, too. Two women – also nurses – who have been friends with Noela for forty-five years won't speak to her. They can't believe her stupidity.

Noela's nursing career may be in tatters but she has many allies in her parallel life, working in alternative health. She uses aromatherapy and massage and is trained in an essential oil practice called Symphony of the Cells™. By her estimation, as many as 90 per cent of practitioners in this 'natural world' have shunned the coronavirus vaccines.

Maureen and Judy are Noela's fellow travellers in the alternative health universe. Maureen worked for years as a medical herbalist, prescribing predominantly Western herbal concoctions from her suburban house until she quit full-time work a decade ago to care for her ailing mother. And Judy – a self-described 'dabbler' in alternative therapies, including healing touch, a Reiki-like therapy with no scientific backing – works as an aged care advocate. Judy says that it's not uncommon for nurses and others in the healthcare and caring industries to become sceptical of the Western approach to healthcare. 'You quickly learn that treatments are band-aids,' she said, and realise that 'there's got to be a better way'.

Anti-vax activists are adept at tapping into the antipathy many feel towards Western medicine. Vaccines are presented as poisonous chemical cocktails that cause untold harms – often covered up, in their view, by an unholy alliance of power-hungry governments and profit-hungry pharmaceutical companies. Better to rely on the body's own natural immune defences, they say.

Julie Leask told me that the 'back to nature' narrative is as old as vaccination itself. In 1885, William White, the first editor of *Vaccination Inquirer*, the journal of the London Society for the Abolition of Compulsory Vaccination, wrote an entire book against vaccination, *The Story of a Great Delusion in a Series of Matter-of-Fact Chapters*. In it, he described vaccination as 'an attempt to swindle nature'.[12] Surprisingly little has changed in the 135-plus years that have elapsed since White's book was published. The diseases and vaccines are different, the arguments against vaccination have evolved, but the underlying themes are identical.

Anti-vaxxers also share common ground with the environmental movement, a traditional concern of the left side of politics. Multinational petrochemical companies pollute waterways and the very air we breathe, just as Big Pharma is seen to be needlessly polluting our bodies. The pursuit of wellness emphasises what the body can do for itself, through good diet and yoga, just as nature would take care of itself if fossil fuel–burning, habitat-encroaching, polluting humans would allow it.

As the COVID-19 vaccines were rolled out, Facebook profile picture frames emblazoned with 'I TRUST MY IMMUNE SYSTEM' proliferated. As did the oft-repeated idea that the only people who die from COVID-19 are people with other conditions to begin with. As Noela sees it, the coronavirus vaccines are the preserve of the elderly and infirm. 'These vaccinations were designed for the elderly and vulnerable, and only for the elderly and the vulnerable,' she told me. For everyone else, she believed, a good dose of vitamin D, vitamin C, zinc and chicken broth should boost the immune system sufficiently, just as they have done for past colds and flus.

But the view of COVID-19 as a disease of the already sick is simply not borne out in the data. It's a sad truth that many people who die of COVID-19 have other chronic illnesses. Indeed, data released by the Australian Bureau of Statistics for COVID-19 deaths that occurred up until the end of January 2022 showed that just shy of 70 per cent of deaths were in people with underlying health conditions. But those conditions did not kill these people. The vast majority of deaths – some 97 per cent – were due directly to COVID-19.[13] Had COVID-19 not come knocking, thousands of people – grandfathers with diabetes, beloved aunts with heart disease, irreplaceable parents with cancer – would have gone on to live fulfilling lives in their communities. They didn't die *with* COVID-19, as Judy argued. They died *from* COVID-19.

On 8 December 2021, Judy tested positive for COVID-19. Two days later, she developed chest pains – a 'red alert' she'd been warned about – and was hauled off to hospital in an ambulance. When a doctor at the hospital gave her the all-clear to leave later that day, he told her, 'You could be just anyone off the street.' I imagine the doctor intended the comment as reassurance: she would be fine. Judy knew how it meant, but it rankled with her nevertheless. 'I thought, "No, I couldn't, I'm very healthy and fit!"' She would later put the whole hospitalisation episode down to stress and having succumbed to the fear-inducing suggestions of medical professionals. Her sense of smell and taste still hadn't returned two months later.

Judy's attitude reminded me of something Katie Attwell, a political scientist at the University of Western Australia, had told me. In pre-COVID times, researchers trying to understand why people harbour scepticism – or outright opposition – towards vaccines focused their attentions on parents. Attwell, whose work looks at the vaccination views of dozens of parents, told me that among parents who refuse vaccinations for their children, some describe their child as being too healthy to need vaccines. In these parents' eyes, their heavily nurtured child – who was breastfed longer than usual, runs around outside in nature, plays with wooden toys, doesn't watch TV, eats organic food and attends the local Steiner school – is fundamentally different from other children. Other kids might need to be vaccinated. Not theirs.

This sort of health exceptionalism was on full display in tennis player Novak Djokovic's remarks after he was denied entry into Australia to defend his tenth title at the Australian Open in January 2022. In an interview with the BBC's Amol Rajan, Djokovic said that he would rather forgo future competitions – and the chance to become the most successful male tennis player of all time – than capitulate to vaccination requirements. 'The principles of decision making on my body are more important than any title or anything else,' he said in the interview, citing his long-standing adherence to 'wellness, wellbeing, health, nutrition' as fundamental to his on-court athleticism. 'I'm trying to be in tune with my body as much as I possibly can.'

For Maureen, vaccines are yet another item in a long list of chemicals that people are unwittingly exposed to. 'We're being bombarded,' she said, with everything from environmental contaminants to additives and pesticide residue on the foods we consume. 'Many years ago, there was DDT, there was thalidomide. God knows what they're putting in our water – fluoride, all that stuff. We don't know what's coming at us.'

Some of the biggest names in the anti-vax world – Joseph Mercola, Larry Cook, Sherri Tenpenny, Rashid Buttar, Sayer Ji, Kelly Brogan, to name a few – are alternative health practitioners or entrepreneurs who earn big bucks selling supplements and alternative health treatments and publishing alternative health news. Their anti-vax messages frequently play on the themes of body purity and 'nature knows best' to sway people concerned about vaccination away from getting vaccinated. Instead, they recommend unproven treatments and supplements – frequently sold on their own websites. Not only do these treatments earn them big money, but they also serve to reinforce the narrative that COVID-19 isn't as bad as the media and government agencies make it out to be, and is easily treatable.

In Australia, the TGA is usually swift to act on unsubstantiated claims about products said to cure COVID-19. Pete Evans, the celebrity chef turned conspiracy theorist and former host of the Channel Seven show *My Kitchen Rules*, started flogging his BioCharger – a device described on his website as a 'hybrid subtle energy revitalisation platform' – when Australia was still in the grip of its first COVID-19 wave. On 9 April 2020, Evans promoted the kitchen blender–sized appliance during a Facebook livestream to his more than 1.4 million followers. 'It's programmed with a thousand different recipes,' he told his viewers. He didn't have time to go into all the details about how the device works, he said, but 'there's a couple in there for Wuhan coronavirus'. People could purchase a BioCharger from Evans' website for the princely sum of $15,000.

Two weeks later, the TGA fined Pete Evans' company $25,200 for his claims about the BioCharger. Thirteen months later, the TGA slapped Evans' company with a further $80,000 in fines for continuing to advertise products purporting to be therapeutic.

Facebook permanently banned Evans from its platform in December 2020. Instagram followed in February 2021. You can still find him on Telegram, though – something which 56,000 of his followers have done. That figure is only 4 per cent of the following he had on Facebook when he promoted his BioCharger, but it's still significant.

While researching this book, I spent an inordinate amount of time in the rabbit warrens of Facebook's alternative health and anti-vaccine mandate pages. I couldn't tell you how I got there, but one of the pages I landed on was for the Health Australia Party. This small Australian political party was co-founded in 2015 by homeopath Isaac Golden. When I spoke with Golden at the start of February 2022, he said that he's very careful about the information he publishes. 'If you look at my website at all, you'll see there is not one word mentioning COVID,' he told me. 'If I mentioned COVID on the webpage, I could be put out of business by the TGA.'

But on the Health Australia Party Facebook page, Golden offers up his wisdom via videos with canary-yellow slides, his earnest face in the bottom corner. There he extols the many natural therapies he claims are 'safe, proven, effective' treatments for COVID-19. On 12 January 2022, for example, his video message offered his 'simple solution' to the COVID-19 hospital crisis caused by surging cases of the Omicron variant. The simple solution: early treatment. Golden directs his viewers to virtual conferences where doctors recommend that people with COVID-19 treat themselves by inhaling hydrogen peroxide, a bleaching agent, and taking high doses of vitamins and zinc. He directs people to papers on hydroxychloroquine and suggests using ivermectin. Both drugs have been embraced by COVID-19 conspiracy theorists and anti-vax activists but universally abandoned as potential treatments by the medical mainstream because they have repeatedly failed in clinical trials.

'The fact that orthodox doctors are not allowed to freely use them in this country is not only a tragedy, it's a scandal,' Golden told me.

Noela has a stash of ivermectin, which she jokingly referred to as her 'horse tablets', for its common use in horse de-worming paste. During the Delta surge in winter 2021, she and her husband took the drug together for a week as a preventive measure. They took it again for a couple of days when her son and his fiancée arrived from the UK in December and caught COVID-19. Neither Noela nor her husband got sick. If they do catch COVID-19, Noela has a recipe for making her own hydroxychloroquine, too.

The enthusiasm for ivermectin and hydroxychloroquine surprised me. It seemed completely at odds with the natural therapy bent of the alternative health industry. Matthew Hornsey, the social psychologist at the University of Queensland, told me that the people drawn to the wellness and alternative medicine scene aren't necessarily all-in on the remedies the industry serves up. Rather, the key connection between that world and vaccine scepticism is the lack of trust. Alternative medicine is their refuge from

Western medicine, from its reliance on mood-altering antidepressants and toxic chemotherapy. Complementary or integrative health is a safer alternative, they believe, and one that doesn't carry with it the taint of Big Pharma.

That's probably why Golden runs a line familiar in antivax rhetoric that's directed at an alternative health–inclined audience. The public is being deceived, he says, because of vested interests. 'Unfortunately, the people who are running the health bureaucracies are totally in cahoots with the pharmaceutical drug cartels,' he told me. Promotion of vaccines over other treatments is an egregious and targeted effort by 'people from chief health officers down' to convince politicians that vaccination is the only way forward. All else is unscientific and unacceptable. Most people who don't do their own research, he said, just accept that narrative.

It's easy to see how people take the next step: from mistrusting pharmaceutical companies and government health agencies, to mistrusting the 'establishment' more broadly. Comments on the Health Australia Party's Facebook page sound like any you might find on sites dedicated to conspiracy theories. 'THE FDA AND TGA ARE ALL PART OF THE NEW WORLD ORDER', shouts one. 'All governments worldwide are puppets of the world economy [sic] forum and they don't want us to know the truth and its [sic] a crime against humanity', reads another. The general vibe of many comments on the page is that people who take the vaccine are coerced, or asleep at the wheel of a vehicle careening towards totalitarianism.

Sociologists Charlotte Ward and David Voas first wrote about the cosy relationship between the belief in conspiracy theories and the New Age in 2011, coining the term 'conspirituality' to describe it.[14] And writers in Australia and elsewhere have noted the disconcerting overlap between the wellness industry and outlandish conspiracies, including QAnon.

As far as I know, Maureen's vaccine scepticism doesn't extend to QAnon, but her ideas read like a playbook of all the worst pandemic conspiracies that have circulated over the past two years. And her fears were depressingly familiar to me, as I'd heard snippets of most from my own mother. The virus doesn't exist. The PCR tests are wrong. The vaccines contain tracking devices. The boosters give you AIDS. She wondered aloud at one point whether there had been a 'mass hypnosis' over COVID-19, which would explain why so many people couldn't see the self-evident truth that she could.

The trio were completely convinced of the truth of their insights into the hidden workings of society that the pandemic had revealed to them: the plots and machinations of those in power, and the corruption and lies that the rest of us were oblivious to or, worse, too fearful to acknowledge to ourselves. History would show that they were on the side of the brave truth-seekers, and they were ready to support them as best as they knew how.

6.
MY BODY, MY CHOICE

In Israel and the UK, people saw the promise of the long-awaited coronavirus vaccines play out in the early months of 2021. Just as officials had predicted, the number of people infected with the virus ebbed as vaccine doses flowed into their arms. Hospitalisations and deaths fell away and the virus receded. Then came the Delta variant, which proved both more contagious and deadlier than previous strains. Along with it came the jarring realisation that COVID-19 was not yet done with us. Numbers climbed once more.

In Australia and New Zealand, the vaccine rollout had a slower start. By the time vaccination was freely available to all adults who wanted it in late August 2021, Delta had arrived in Australia, and its rampant spread had plunged more than half of the country's population into lockdown.

Governments around the country clung to a zero-COVID policy, which was no match for Delta. Lockdowns chafed at the nerves of an exhausted population, demoralised after two years of restrictions, and by the curve's stubborn refusal to flatten back to zero.

Unable to staunch the virus's spread, and with vaccine supply now largely meeting demand, authorities focused on vaccination targets. A complicated matrix of targets and restrictions that varied from state to state had nearly all eyes glued to vaccination rates, which crept incrementally higher as August turned into September, then October and November.

Focus also shifted to vaccination mandates. The first COVID-19 vaccine mandate introduced in Australia was in the private sector. In August 2021, the fruit-canning company SPC mandated COVID-19 vaccination for the 450 staff at its Shepparton-based cannery, and any visitors to the site. Government mandates started kicking in not long after. In the final half of 2021, states around Australia enacted vaccine mandates. Mandates for healthcare workers, for aged care workers, for teachers and childcare workers, and, in Victoria, for almost any worker unable to work from home.

History makes a compelling argument for vaccine mandates. In 1806, when Napoleon Bonaparte was charging his armies across Europe and declaring his brother, Joseph, King of Spain, his sister Elisa – who ruled a small principality in modern-day Tuscany – was making history as the first European leader to mandate vaccination.

Babies within two months of their birth and all adults were required to be vaccinated against smallpox using the cowpox vaccination method discovered by Englishman Edward Jenner a decade earlier.

Over the next few years, vaccination against smallpox was heavily promoted throughout the Napoleonic Kingdom in northern Italy. Funding, government bureaucracies, vaccination decrees and what we would today recognise as 'no jab, no pay' and 'no jab, no play' laws proliferated. By 1813, Francesco Cornalia, prefect of Serio, declared that smallpox – 'a monster that committed much slaughter and caused many other dreadful effects' – had disappeared. That assessment was, sadly, a touch on the optimistic side. But the campaign was judged a success – it's estimated that more than one million people in the Napoleonic Kingdom, primarily children, were vaccinated over a twelve-year period, and thousands of lives were spared.[15]

Across nineteenth-century Europe, stark differences in smallpox rates emerged between regions where mandates were adopted and those where they were not. A tenfold higher death rate from the disease in England and Wales, compared to places such as Italy (where mandates operated), convinced authorities to introduce a mandate in 1853. When Germany mandated smallpox vaccination in 1874, deaths plummeted thirty-fold, a fall that neighbouring countries without mandates missed out on.

With mandates came anti-mandate protests and activists. In Britain, the Anti-Compulsory Vaccination League was founded in London in 1866, just thirteen years after a mandate was enacted. By 1871 its membership had mushroomed to 10,000 people across 103 separate branches, and in 1896 it joined forces with other groups around the country, forming the National Anti-Vaccination League. Anti-vaccination organisations in Britain and similar groups in North America lobbied governments, published anti-vaccination pamphlets and journals, and organised protests. In 1885, a massive demonstration in Leicester, England, reportedly attracted more than 80,000 people. Angry protesters marched through the streets, waving banners, and brandishing an effigy of Edward Jenner and a child's coffin.

Fast-forward to November 2021, when the Austrian government announced it would make COVID-19 vaccination mandatory for everyone aged eighteen years and older. From 1 February 2022, those unwilling to be vaccinated would be fined. Until that point, countries had wielded mandates as a protective measure only in certain settings. Mandates for healthcare and aged care workers were enacted across Europe, the US, Canada, New Zealand, Latin America and elsewhere. As the Omicron wave began to swell, governments around the world sought to expand mandates to other sectors. To teachers, firefighters, police and government employees. Private companies also turned to mandates, to protect their workforce, their customers and their liability. Governments and private industry imposed restrictions that reached beyond the workforce to the unvaxxed entering shops and entertainment venues, eateries and sporting arenas.

At every turn, mandates were supported by the majority and railed against by a vocal, sometimes violent minority.

Close to 95 per cent of Australians aged sixteen and over are vaccinated against COVID-19. But it's almost impossible – frustratingly so – to figure out whether we would have got where we are without vaccine mandates. In Austria, an additional 5.5 per cent of the population received at least one dose of vaccine in the three months following the announcement of the population-wide mandate. But the number still only topped out at 75.2 per cent of the total population. In Australia, the population-level number is close to 86 per cent.

Almost every expert that I spoke to about vaccine mandates – from epidemiologists and psychologists, to social scientists and bioethicists – prevaricated when asked whether vaccine mandates are justified.

That's because there is no clear answer. You can't put the data into a machine and crank a handle to find out if the answer is forty-two. It will always depend. It will depend on how bad the outbreak is, how well the vaccine protects you from disease, how well it protects others from infection, and what level of fallout the community is willing to bear. It's also a political calculation. Mandates are popular, and play well at both ends of the political spectrum, from the law-and-order advocates on the right to the public health and civic responsibility–minded left.

Omicron has made the question of vaccine mandates even thornier. Within a few weeks of lockdowns easing, kids returning to school and interstate borders (except for Western Australia) reopening, Omicron was upon us, dwarfing the outbreaks that came before it. The Omicron variant is even more contagious than the already hard-to-contain Delta. And while it is thankfully less severe, its oddball mix of mutations allows it to evade immunity gained from exposure to previous strains, as well as from the available vaccines, which were all designed against much earlier versions of the virus. In other words, you can still catch Omicron, even if you've diligently bared your fleshy upper arm for the recommended two doses plus a booster shot.

These factors all fed into the anti-vax narrative that the vaccines don't work, that COVID-19 is less severe than authorities claim, and that getting vaccinated is an 'all risk, no gain' proposition, because people who are vaccinated are no better off.

Those claims are false, even with the advent of Omicron. In January 2022, at the peak of the Omicron outbreak, the small percentage of people who remained unvaxxed – not counting young children and others ineligible for the vaccine – were over-represented among COVID-19 casualties. They accounted for 18 per cent of COVID-19 cases overall, nearly half of those who ended up in hospital (45 per cent), and nearly two-thirds of those who ended up in the intensive care unit (62 per cent). Most chillingly, they represented half of those who died. Data from the US Centers for Disease Control and Prevention estimated that in January 2022 – amid the surge in Omicron cases – an unvaccinated person was nine times more likely to die of COVID-19 than someone who's had two shots, and twenty-one times more likely to die than someone who's been 'boosted' with a third shot.[16]

Omicron has challenged the general public's understanding of vaccines and what we can rightly expect from them. The common view of vaccines is that when they work, they prevent infection. And by preventing infection in enough people you eliminate the opportunity for a virus to bounce through the population from one person to the next, to the next, to the next, and voila! You've achieved herd immunity. The truth so many of us have now become familiar with is that some vaccines – the coronavirus vaccines, yes, but also the whooping cough vaccine and flu vaccines – are 'leaky'. They don't stop the contagion in its tracks by preventing people from being infected and from passing it on. Even the fully vaccinated can, on occasion, spread the illness to others, especially the unvaxxed.

But it's not an all-or-nothing proposition. Catherine Bennett, an infectious diseases epidemiologist from Deakin University who has become a familiar face during the pandemic, laid out a hypothetical when we spoke. She said that people who have been vaccinated with two doses are only two-thirds as likely to catch Omicron compared with someone who is unvaxxed. So, instead of 45,000 cases, you'd only have 30,000 cases. Give everyone a third booster shot and the risk of infection is halved again. Now you've only got 15,000 cases. And fewer people getting infected means fewer people ending up in hospital, in ICU wards and on ventilators. Instead of 300 on ventilators, perhaps you only have 100. 'That's huge!' she said.

Bennett told me that considering how vastly different Omicron is to previously circulating variants, it's remarkable that the vaccines protect us as much as they do. And given how well they protect against the strange, wildly divergent beast that is Omicron, odds are that our arsenal (if we've had our three shots) is well stocked against the next variant that will, inevitably, come along.

Regardless, Omicron has left many – including governments around the world – questioning the merits of vaccine mandates. In the UK, plans for vaccine mandates for health staff were abandoned at the end of January 2022. I spoke to Dominic Wilkinson, a medical ethicist at the University of Oxford, about the decision. He told me that the case for vaccine mandates fell apart with Omicron because fully vaccinated healthcare workers can still transmit the virus, because the virus is less harmful, and because alternatives, in the form of personal protective equipment, are available. In the UK, the decision was made that the mandate was no longer a proportional measure given the gains it would provide.

When I spoke to Katie Attwell from the University of Western Australia, she told me that mandates rarely convince vaccine refusers to change their mind. Mandates exist primarily to increase vaccine uptake, thereby reducing the general risk of disease through widespread immunity.

But they won't turn a trenchant objector into a vaccine acceptor. What they can do, she said, is nudge the people who are still mulling over the decision, who would prefer to 'wait a while' because they are hesitant, to take the plunge sooner rather than later. Considering the weeks spent in lockdown obsessively waiting for the vaccination trigger point for reopening to be reached, it's easy to see the value in that.

But mandates also run the risk of nudging people who are unsure about the vaccine towards outright refusal. On top of that, mandates have the power to polarise the community, and radicalise people who feel unjustly punished for their decision not to get vaccinated. Mandates can also galvanise people against vaccination and cause a backlash against other vaccines.

Each time a state announced a vaccine mandate in the closing months of 2021, a run of stories in the media predicted how many workers might lose their jobs, and how short-staffed a particular sector might be once the mandate took effect. Final tallies of how many workers do end up quitting or being fired are less easy to track down. But from the few numbers that are reported, it appears that only a tiny number of workers – usually 1 per cent or less – are willing to lose their jobs rather than be vaccinated. In New South Wales, for instance, just 125 full-time teachers and one principal were stood down by the Department of Education and a further 334 decided to leave their jobs. That's well under 1 per cent of the state's nearly 80,000 public school teachers.

In Western Australia, the Department of Education expected to lose about 300 teachers – or just 1 per cent – due to the mandate. By mid-January 2022, only 995 of NSW Health's 170,000-strong workforce – or a smidgen north of half a per cent – had resigned or been stood down after refusing the vaccine.

After two years during which parts of Australia were locked down and others awaited the return of interstate and international travel, many were outraged at anyone not willing to do their part. On 22 November 2021, the Australian Senate rejected a bill introduced by One Nation that would have toppled state health orders requiring employees, patrons at bars and cafés, retail customers, students, gym- and concert-goers, and guests at hotels to be vaccinated. Independent senator Jacqui Lambie slapped down the bill and its framing as an anti-discrimination measure ahead of the vote. 'If you're able to get vaccinated, and you choose not to, discrimination is the wrong word,' she said. 'Being held accountable for your own actions isn't called discrimination, it's called being, you wouldn't believe it, a goddamn bloody adult,' she blasted, channelling the rage that people across the nation were feeling. 'It's putting others before yourself. And that's what this country is supposed to be about.'

One Nation adopted the language of discrimination in its bill. But anti-vax activists adopted the language of the pro-choice movement: 'My body, my choice'. Still others, hitching their wagon to the growing discontent, used the language of autonomy: mandates aren't about public health, they are about personal freedom.

When I asked Matthew Hornsey from the University of Queensland about his view on mandates, he wasn't sure how to answer. But he summed up the conundrum that governments around the world are still grappling with. 'The question is, what's the biggest cost to society? Because I think it does work, it gets people vaccinated at the end of the day,' he said. 'And so if the public health crisis is critical enough, maybe it's worth doing.'

Julie Leask told me that mandates should be a last resort, because the downsides of mandating vaccines are substantial. 'If you're just getting marginal protection from a requirement versus other measures,' she said, 'it's probably not worth it'.

Was the health crisis critical enough? Is it still? That calculation will need to be made again and again, as it has for lockdowns and masks and indoor gatherings and events. But governments need to beware the backlash that comes with asking that people decide between their principles and their livelihoods, because the cost could well spill out beyond lives lost to COVID-19.

7.
SOWING DIVISIONS

For Maureen, one of the trio I spoke with on the Port Phillip foreshore, the experiences of the past year have been personally shattering. Her husband got fully vaccinated with two shots before she found out. When her husband's vaccinations came to light, she implored him to let her know next time he decided to get a shot, so that she could take precautions to protect herself from the spike proteins that he would shed, genuinely fearful that her vaccinated husband might make her sick. He went and got the booster without telling her anyway. They remain together, but the rift has shaken her. Her once sturdy relationship has turned icy. 'I feel like I'm living with an alien,' she said.

Her daughter-in-law's family have also snubbed her. When she went to the auction of her son's house, his mother-in-law told her, 'Don't come near me. You've been to the protest, and you've got unvaccinated friends, and with all due respect, I don't want you to come anywhere near me.' Maureen was devastated.

After Judy got COVID-19 in December 2021, she got a medical exemption from her doctor. Having been infected with the virus, she was considered immune, and for the next six months she doesn't have to worry about getting vaccinated. She's waiting to see what happens with the vaccine developed by Nikolai Petrovsky and his South Australian company Vaxine, or perhaps she'll get COVID-19 again. 'That might help me out,' she says. Before she got her exemption, Judy said she could 'feel the discrimination'. Casual acquaintances would visibly recoil from her when it came up in conversation. 'It puts you in the shoes of the refugees, I suppose, or the Indigenous,' she said.

'We've had two years of COVID, and the first year without the jab, we were all equal,' Noela said, 'and since the jabs have come in, it's segregated'. In her bag, Noela has her 'illegal little piece of paper', a fake vaccine certificate she downloaded online, so she doesn't miss out. 'I've got my normal freedoms that were my freedoms before this,' she says.

A few days before I met them, Judy and Noela had attended a meeting of the AustraliaOne Party, one of a handful of fledgling conservative or right-leaning political parties gaining traction in online communities opposed to vaccine mandates and other pandemic restrictions. Riccardo Bosi, the leader of AustraliaOne, lists the intentions of his yet-to-be-registered political party on his LinkedIn profile. 'Purpose: To Save Australia', he writes. Further down he lists the 'Endstate', being that 'Australia is a moral, sovereign, self-reliant Christian western democracy, which is: economically powerful; militarily intimidating; politically free; culturally vibrant; socially cohesive'.

Judy, who was at the time active in a local left-leaning campaign for an independent candidate at the upcoming federal election, was still reeling from what she'd heard at the meeting. The crowd of Frankston locals was rowdy and uncouth, not what the women were accustomed to. But Judy was ready to listen and learn.

Speaking at the event was Craig Cole, the party's state coordinator for Victoria. As she listened, Judy tried to weigh the group's merits – Cole spoke of transparency and corruption – against what she recognised as clear falsehoods (laws allowing full-term abortions, for instance) and bizarre claims she couldn't quite place. 'I'd like to know about the paedophilia thing,' she mused. I can only guess that Cole perhaps referred to QAnon-type conspiracies about global elites running secret child-trafficking and paedophile rings. The group's opposition to vaccine mandates had bridged a gap that I would have thought unbridgeable. It was unfathomable that someone like Judy – engaged in local grassroots political processes to bolster action on climate change – had crossed so far as to be casually curious about conspiracies associated with QAnon and the alt-right. It bothered me that others might likewise find their curiosity piqued.

At the end of January 2022, protesters against vaccine mandates converged on Canberra, travelling to the capital from all over the east coast of Australia. Noela saw Bosi speak online in broadcasts from the Canberra protests as they were heating up, and was impressed by what she saw. She was also impressed by Mark Latham, though she couldn't immediately place which party he belongs to (it's the conservative One Nation Party). 'I quite like his views on a lot of people,' she said.

I asked whether the rightward slant of AustraliaOne was a departure from what I had assumed to be a left-leaning proclivity in the alternative health world. That wasn't the case for Noela. 'Coming from natural therapies, etc. and medical backgrounds, well, I have never ever been interested in politics,' she said.

That's all changed. Vaccine mandates have galvanised her to become politically engaged for the first time in her life. Noela's concerns about freedoms curtailed by vaccine mandates have eclipsed all other issues that might have determined her vote at the ballot box. 'My situation at the moment is, I want someone to question these mandates. I want someone to stand up and say, well is that right or not?' she said. 'I mean, climate change to me …' she trailed off with a shrug. Climate change posed no immediate threat; vaccine mandates were a clear and present danger. 'I want people to change this world that we're living in at the moment, because the world's turned on its axis. If you asked me, I can't believe the situation has got so out of hand.'

And now, in the 2022 federal election, she's considering sending her vote to political parties that have seen their popularity mushroom because of the discontent of the now trenchant objectors like Noela.

As the country lurched through its first pandemic year in 2020, community resolve to fight the virus started to wane, and frustrations boiled over. Lockdowns and travel restrictions, and the devastating personal and financial toll these measures were taking, left many questioning the high price of controlling what they felt was an intangible viral bogeyman. Melbourne, encircled by a metaphorical 'Ring of Steel' that kept city-dwellers from travelling to regional Victoria, became a hotbed for discontent during a months-long lockdown. In September, hundreds marched for their 'freedom', and in November, hundreds more were spritzed with capsicum spray and arrested.

But 2021 was the year that the situation turned truly ugly. Protests spread across the country and anti-lockdown 'freedom rallies' quickly took up the cudgels against mandatory vaccination rules that were being applied to a growing number of industries. In September 2021, violence erupted at a protest against mandatory vaccination for construction workers. Dan Andrews' state government responded by slapping the industry with a snap two-week closure. Protests raged for several more days.

Amid the chaos and rancour, questions of who was behind the protests – in 2020, 2021, and now in 2022 – have swirled. Many have pointed the finger at right-wing agitators and conspiracy-minded anarchist groups. But pinpointing who was attending – let alone organising – the rallies is a fraught endeavour.

Protest leaders linked to right-wing organisations, including the international white supremacist group the Proud Boys, have been blamed for fomenting some of the 2020 protests. And in May 2021, the data science organisation Logically traced 129 global anti-lockdown and anti-vax protests to a group based in the German town of Kassel. 'Freie Bürger Kassel', or the Free Citizens of Kassel, spouts COVID-19 conspiracy theories as well as anti-vax and Islamophobic messages through a global network under the 'World Wide Demonstration' banner.[17] That same group instigated lockdown protests across Australia in July 2021, including large demonstrations in Sydney and Melbourne, according to an investigation by *The Guardian*.[18]

At the Canberra Convoy, prominent conservative and right-leaning politicians including the LNP's George Christensen, One Nation's Pauline Hanson and United Australia Party's Craig Kelly all made appearances in support of the anti-vaccine protests. They were joined by self-styled freedom-fighting activists and grassroots anti-vax groups like Parents With Questions. In New Zealand, too, pro-Trump flags rippled in the wind on the lawns in front of the 'Beehive' parliament building in Wellington, as thousands gathered to decry the nation's vaccine mandates. On 3 March 2022, the three-week long protest ended with New Zealand police towing vehicles away and dismantling the protesters' encampment. Demonstrators lit fires fuelled by abandoned mattresses and tents.

Katie Attwell is worried. She said that anti-vax rallies of the pre-COVID era attracted a very different crowd. Most would have been progressive-leaning mothers who identified as feminists. With COVID-19, she said, there's been 'a big fat injection of toxicity from the alt-right', which has been imported from places like the US. She told me of a colleague who attended an anti-mandate rally in Perth. One man at the rally wore a T-shirt emblazoned with the words 'Feminism is cancer', a slogan associated with the alt-right. Few at the protest may have shared those views, but Attwell worries that groups with particular agendas are edging their way into anti-vax circles to reach a new audience, drawing them in to a populist style of politics that has polarised Americans. It's a prospect Attwell finds incredibly frightening.

Stephan Lewandowsky has similar concerns. 'The extreme right has instrumentalised, well, ... everything. Vaccinations, social restrictions, mask wearing.' He told me that groups active before the pandemic have opportunistically glommed onto pandemic discontent, and have now galvanised around the opposition to vaccine mandates. 'All they want is to create anti-government sentiment and division in society, because that's what they thrive on,' he said.

Aleksandra Cichocka, who runs the political psychology lab at the University of Kent in the UK, says that her native Poland is a cautionary tale in how populist politics can go awry. Poland is among a handful of countries that have lurched rightwards in recent years. In 2015, the right-leaning Law & Justice Party – which ran on an anti-elite platform not dissimilar to Donald Trump's 'drain the swamp' bombast – was unexpectedly successful at the polls. Since then, the party has fanned a conspiratorial worldview in the country, and a mistrust in authority. For instance, the Law & Justice Party's chairman and co-founder, Jarosław Kaczyński, promotes a false narrative about the 2010 air crash that killed ninety-six people – including his twin brother, the then-president of Poland, Lech Kaczyński – as a political assassination orchestrated by the Russian government.

In this climate, vaccine scepticism flourished. During the party's first five years in government from 2015, vaccine refusal grew threefold, according to Poland's National Health Institute. In the July 2020 elections, with vaccines still months away, the Polish president, Andrzej Duda, openly courted the anti-vaxxer vote, promising there would be no mandate introduced for a COVID-19 vaccine when one became available. The surge in vaccine refusal has hit hard during COVID-19. 'Putting everybody in that conspiratorial mindset is backfiring massively,' Cichocka told me. Poland's vaccine rollout lags behind the European Union average and had almost completely stalled at 59 per cent of the population at the end of February 2022. The final 10 per cent of that was eked out over more than six months.

Among the crowds in Canberra were people not dissimilar to Noela and Judy and Maureen. People who were attending the protest less out of political affiliation than a desire to protect their decision to remain unvaxxed. They wanted to be with others who felt the same, and with people willing to fight for a cause that barely existed in their minds prior to the pandemic but is now central to who they are. What those people found was camaraderie and community. But they would have also brushed shoulders with people equating mandates to an irrevocable erosion of democracy, a slide towards totalitarianism, a re-run of Nazism and worse.

People reluctant, and now determined, not to take the new COVID-19 vaccines would have come across people like Meryl Dorey from the Australian Vaccination-risks Network, who shun all vaccines, not just the new COVID-19 shots. Dorey was jubilant as she drove through the crowd in the group's 'Vaxxed Bus' – fashioned after the 2016 movie of the same name directed by anti-vax activist Andrew Wakefield – ready to film testimonials from parents of children apparently injured by vaccines.

Matthew Hornsey told me that antipathy towards vaccination shows up at both extremes of the political spectrum. Belief in conspiracy theories – which hinge on deep-seated mistrust in government and established institutions – follows a similar trend. In the hodge-podge of the anti-mandate rallies, where populist notions of freedom and democracy and personal choice are shouted from lecterns, it may be a smaller sidestep than we might imagine to traverse the political spectrum from left-leaning greenie to the QAnon-curious anti-government conspiracy world that has become the mainstay of the American alt-right.

Given the structure of the Australian political system, small slivers of the electorate can have a bigger influence than their raw numbers suggest. It's hard to know from the outside what motivates politicians like George Christensen – who is not planning to recontest his seat at the upcoming election – and Craig Kelly, who jumped ship from the Liberal Party to become leader of the United Australia Party. Should their strong anti-vax stance be cynically viewed as a ploy to gain an audience, to win votes? How sincere are they? And how much will support from disaffected voters like Noela affect the Australian political landscape?

8.
WHAT NEXT?

On 1 February 2022, Denmark declared the pandemic over. The Scandinavian nation scrapped most of its remaining COVID-19 restrictions – mask-wearing orders, border controls and vaccination passes were dropped. COVID-19 is no longer classified as a 'socially critical disease'. The Danish prime minister, Mette Frederiksen, made no promises that this will always be the case. 'I dare not say that it is a final goodbye to restrictions,' she said. But for now, life is returning to something resembling what it was before the pandemic struck.

Elsewhere, too, restrictions are easing. From the beginning of February, travellers to the European Union could enter with or without vaccination, no matter where they had travelled from. If unvaxxed, a negative test result would suffice. Vaccination rates across the European Union sit on a sliding scale, from 94 per cent in Portugal and Malta to just 59 per cent in Poland. By the end of the same month, the UK prime minister, Boris Johnson, had set out a plan for 'living with COVID', which included dropping the recommendation for certain venues to check vaccination status from 1 April. Seventy-nine per cent of the UK's sixty-seven million people are vaccinated. And New Zealand – 87 per cent vaccinated – will open its borders to unvaccinated visitors in April, provided they quarantine upon arrival.

In Australia – also 87 per cent vaccinated – state-based COVID-19 restrictions remain but are gradually falling away. International borders, controlled at the federal level, have opened to people who have been vaccinated, or are exempt from vaccination. No announcements have been made about when unvaccinated travellers will be allowed to enter the country.

Pandemic deniers and minimisers have repeatedly compared COVID-19 to the flu, or a 'bad cold'. Now experts are also making that comparison, given the nature of Omicron, and the widespread immunity stemming from vaccination and to a lesser extent past infections. Even so, there is no telling what COVID-19 has in store for us. More than half the world's seven billion people have received at least one dose of a COVID-19 vaccine, but large swathes of the developing world await the arrival of even their first dose of protection. This is something that should concern us all. As long as the virus continues to circulate – and it will circulate far more freely in the unvaccinated – we will continue to work our way through the Greek alphabet of new variants. They won't necessarily be milder, despite the false assertion by anti-vaxxers that viruses always tend towards milder versions over time. We've already seen that happen with Delta, which was both more contagious than previously circulating variants, and more likely to land someone in hospital if they caught it. The BA.2 subvariant of Omicron is already gaining ground, replacing the original subvariant of Omicron, BA.1, as the most dominant strain. In Europe, Australia and elsewhere, case numbers are on the rise again. We don't yet know when this wave will crest, nor when – or where – the variant driving the next wave will appear.

The long tail of the COVID-19 pandemic will reach well into the future. Families and friends will carry the grief of loved ones lost to the virus. Others have the lingering aftereffects of long COVID, unable to work or enjoy life as they used to. Young children have missed out on crucial months of learning, socialising and playing at school. Older kids have had to navigate the final, competitive years of schooling alone at their computers. 'For Lease' signs tell a horrifying tale of the businesses – and dreams and livelihoods – that have collapsed. Careers – especially those of women with young children – have been slammed by the extra responsibilities that have come with childcare and home-schooling. And the trauma of it all has come with a devastating cost to the nation's mental health. People are waiting months to see a psychologist. In New South Wales, the number of children turning up at emergency departments having self-harmed jumped by 47 per cent during the pandemic.[19] And nearly two-thirds of the country's performing artists say their mental health has taken a hit.[20] There is no quick fix.

Vaccines were always billed as the way out of the pandemic. That has turned out to be the case. Despite lingering restrictions, despite the arrival of the immune-dodging Omicron variant, and despite the fact that people – both vaxxed and unvaxxed – got sick, ended up in hospital and even died, we wouldn't be where we are now were it not for the vaccines that lessened the viral assault for most of us. That has kept all of us safer – not only from COVID-19, but from the devastation that would have occurred if the health system had collapsed, buckling under the weight of full-blown COVID-19 cases in a completely unvaccinated community.

But how much we now lean on vaccination, and how much we restrict the unvaxxed, is unclear. In Victoria, the Andrews government shelved plans to make a third booster shot compulsory for workers across the state, but only because practicalities got in the way. With international arrivals requiring only two vaccine doses to be fully vaccinated, the three-dose requirement became untenable. 'There comes a point where things become impractical and you've got so many systems operating at once that it doesn't really work,' Premier Dan Andrews said on 16 February 2022.

Omicron has closed the immunity gap. Many unvaccinated people were infected with Omicron over the summer months, and those people are now potentially as immune to reinfection as people who received their booster shot. But they might not be as immune to the next variant that comes along. And immunity for everyone decreases. We won't know until several months out from the Omicron wave how quickly immunity wanes – for those with naturally acquired immunity and for those who have had a booster shot. Nevertheless, fears of pharmaceutical companies capitalising on quarterly booster shots look increasingly unlikely to bear out. A slew of studies on immune protections of a third shot shows that protection against severe illness and death – even if not from infection – could be long lasting. But again, no one knows for sure.

The continuing parade of viral variants will make the immunity picture even messier than it already is. The traditional view of herd immunity – that it stops transmission within the community because susceptible people are too few and far between for the virus to hop around and do damage – is too simplistic. Over time, the community will be filled with people who have been vaccinated at different times, and have different levels of immunity from their first, second and third shots. There will be others who have caught the virus, providing an unknowable level of immunity against the variant they were infected with and against the unknown variants that might come along. On top of that, there will always be some people who can ride out the infection with fewer complications and lingering effects than others.

This all makes the question of how much risk the unvaxxed pose to the rest of us exceedingly difficult to answer. When Novak Djokovic was denied entry into the country in January, it was initially because he did not meet the vaccination requirements needed to enter. A judge overruled the visa cancellation, but Immigration Minister Alex Hawke cancelled the visa again, this time 'on health and good order grounds'. Hawke decided that it was in the public interest to deport Djokovic, not because he was unvaxxed, nor because he had failed to complete his immigration forms correctly, but because he was 'perceived by some as a talisman of a community of anti-vaccine sentiment', according to Hawke. In other words, there was fear that his very presence might incite unrest.

Community outrage was palpable during the fortnight-long Djokovic saga. Australians had spent months in lockdown, isolated from family and friends, home-schooling their children, and watching their businesses and mental health deteriorate. Then, collectively, they had rolled up their sleeves, even those who were still concerned, or who still harboured doubts and anxieties. After all of that, the Australian public had little appetite for someone so brazenly snubbing the rules that everyone else had followed. The question of whether Djokovic posed a danger – in terms of COVID-19, at least – was secondary.

Djokovic isn't the only person to feel the brunt of community outrage over a decision he likely felt was personal – his and his alone to make. On 5 January 2022, *Le Parisien* published an interview with French president Emmanuel Macron. Speaking about the restrictions on the unvaxxed, he said: 'The unvaccinated, I really want to piss them off. And so we're going to continue doing so until the end. That's the strategy.'

Meanwhile, the UK was dealing with its own scandal. In November 2021, it came to light that Boris Johnson, members of his government and Downing Street staff attended parties during periods of lockdown in 2020 and 2021, blatantly flouting the restrictions they themselves had imposed on the country.

With world leaders talking and acting in this way, it's no wonder that people question the motives behind vaccine mandates and other pandemic control measures. Do they keep people safe? Or are they punitive measures?

Throughout the pandemic, politicians of all colours have claimed to be following public health advice and the science that underpins it. Mathematical modelling graphs were wheeled out at press conferences, showing how restrictions would bend an upward curve towards a benign flatline. But mathematical modelling was not a factor in deciding to apply mandates.

Some mandates – such as those covering aged care and frontline healthcare staff – are designed to protect especially vulnerable people from infection. In these cases, calculating their impact on overall transmission rates and case numbers in a population makes little sense, and there is widespread support for vaccine mandates in these settings. A *Guardian* poll in September 2021 – before Omicron came along – found that over 80 per cent of Australians thought mandatory vaccination was a good idea for health and care workers. But those percentages crumbled for other settings: for sporting events, 69 per cent; hospitality venues, 68 per cent; workplaces, 62 per cent; and schools, just 58 per cent.[21]

Broader vaccine mandates – such as the mandate introduced in Victoria that covers most working adults who can't work alone – were introduced to lift vaccine uptake across the population. But they should be proportional to the benefit they provide, and that hasn't been demonstrated. With more than 94 per cent of eligible Australians over the age of sixteen fully vaccinated, the benefit is likely marginal at best, especially with Omicron. In Austria, the government introduced an unprecedented law to fine unvaccinated adults up to €3600 starting in mid-March 2022, but it abandoned the law on 9 March because it was no longer proportional to the threat posed by Omicron.

The unvaxxed are, by far, a minority in Australia, and we shouldn't lose sight of this fact. Most Australians have complied with government restrictions and public health recommendations. They have stayed home, worn masks, got tested with no more than a sniffle, isolated themselves if a friend has gotten sick, and gone out of their way to get vaccinated – not once, not twice, but often three times so far. At the height of the Omicron wave, people stayed home even when no rules required them to. This 'shadow lockdown' shows that people are willing to protect themselves in the absence of population-wide lockdowns and transmission-scuttling vaccines.

There is no easy antidote to vaccine refusal. Indeed, the experts that I spoke to about attitudes to vaccination said that you will never convince everyone to get vaccinated. There will always be the trenchant objectors, as Leask calls them. But there are things that the government can do.

Firstly, as much as humanly possible, wrecking balls need to be taken to any and all access barriers that exist, whether that's a language barrier, a transport barrier, or lack of time or money. Targeted, community-guided interventions can be phenomenally successful. But they take effort and resources to put in place. If people in a community are not coming forward to be vaccinated, vaccination needs to go to them.

The second thing that needs to happen is to limit the influence that trenchant objectors – and even more so, anti-vax activists – have over people who are unsure about vaccination. This isn't a role that the government can take on alone. We all bear responsibility for setting the norms in society to reassure the hesitant and anxious among us. Rolling up our sleeves to prevent vaccine-preventable diseases is one part of that. But vaccination is already the norm. We also need to show consideration and respect for people whose values and experiences and access to information lead them to make decisions at odds with our own. Too often, we succumb to the urge to judge and scold, especially when another person's actions – or inaction – rubs up against our own anxieties. Many people have been rightly fearful about catching COVID-19, and have little patience for others who place them at increased risk of infection.

There might be a handful of people who refuse to get vaccinated because it boosts their personal brand as a misfit or rugged individual who shirks societal norms. But I suspect that most who remain unvaxxed genuinely believe that the decision they are making is the right decision. They are safeguarding their own health, and are anxious about loved ones who are not protecting themselves in the same way. These people deserve our compassion and respect. Dismissing their concerns out of hand serves no one's interests in the long run. Listening – really listening – to peoples' concerns and their root causes shows respect, builds connection, and has the ability to change minds.

The government bears some responsibility, too. On the federal Department of Health's website, there's a page filled with answers to some of the most common concerns about COVID-19 vaccines. On the 'Is it true? Get the facts on COVID-19 vaccines' page, visitors can find answers from the mundane – how long does it take to have immunity after vaccination? – to the more colourful: do the vaccines cause infertility? Or connect you to the internet? Or contain microchips?

At the very bottom of the page, there's also a question about mandates. Are COVID-19 vaccines mandatory in Australia? Click through, and you find an answer that verges on gaslighting. 'Vaccination for COVID-19 is voluntary – as are all vaccinations in Australia – and people maintain the option to choose.' It mentions that residential aged care workers are required to vaccinate, and that 'there may be circumstances in the future in which proof of vaccination will be required, such as border or re-entry requirements, or continued employment in particular areas'. There's no other mention of or links to state-based laws that have generated such upheaval in people's lives, not to mention the protests and rallies and general community unrest.

When governments fail to communicate openly and honestly, trust is the casualty. Open and honest communication extends beyond simply communicating daily case counts and deaths; uncertainty, too, must be conveyed. Governments around the world have struggled to strike a balance in their communications about COVID-19, fearing that they will lose authority if they say they are unsure. A study by researchers at University College London that is yet to be peer-reviewed found that loss of trust was greater when vaccine information was communicated with certainty rather than uncertainty.[22]

In the early weeks of the pandemic, numerous public health officials openly derided the idea of the general public wearing facemasks to staunch the spread of a virus that they were adamant was not airborne. Of course, masks became a staple pandemic control measure, and most countries now have programs in place to increase ventilation to deal with the coronavirus as the airborne contagion that it is.

It's no wonder people question public health advice with such monumental backflips. Communicating uncertainty – 'current evidence suggests that this is the best approach, but advice may change when we learn more', say – prevents the whiplash that people feel when they get conflicting information. Not acknowledging missteps and failing to set up a narrative that explains why the situation is changing and will likely change again undermines trust and plays into fears that there are ulterior motives at work. Anti-vax activists and political opportunists will always capitalise on this, seeking to torpedo trust in vaccination and other policies. Governments should be wary of inadvertently providing fodder for these tactics.

Of course, effective communication can only do so much. New Zealand's prime minister Jacinda Ardern has been widely praised for her style of open and honest communication during the pandemic. At the start, she laid out clear COVID alert levels, indicating when those levels would kick in and what restrictions would be in place when they did. But effective communication can only do so much. But anti-vaccine mandate protests – against targeted vaccination requirements for some workers and vaccine passes to enter most stores and restaurants – took hold in Wellington in February 2022 nonetheless.

There will always be people who make ill-advised decisions that might land them in hospital or in a coffin. The difficulty lies when the consequences of those decisions are borne by everyone. Smokers are able to smoke, but they can't light up wherever they like because their smoke harms the health of others. COVID-19 is often compared to smoking in this respect, as though the unvaxxed issue forth a plume of contagion that will infect the rest of us. But such a simple dichotomy between the vaxxed and the unvaxxed does not exist. There are degrees of infectiousness, degrees of susceptibility. We can rail against the unfairness of people who have shirked their communal responsibility to play their part in putting an end to the pandemic, but we also need to acknowledge the nuances that have emerged with Omicron. The unvaxxed pose a far greater risk to themselves than they do to others at this stage of the pandemic.

The rifts that have opened up over the past year can feel insurmountable. I haven't heard from my mum in months, and I'm pretty certain that she's blocked my mobile number. She may have read the email I sent her recently, but it's possible that she deleted it straightaway, or hasn't even seen it – my brother said she's wary of using her Gmail account because she doesn't want Google to track her. My brother and his kids have moved out of the house they shared, and I imagine she has become even more reliant on the online communities she belongs to than she was before.

I bear some of the responsibility for this. I dismissed her fears, refused to engage with – or even listen to – what she was saying. If I'd listened to her concerns, I might have learned what drew her to her beliefs, and I might have been able to sow a seed of doubt in her mind about the veracity of the information she reads online. Her scepticism about the motivations of government and Big Pharma might have been harnessed to question the motives of people spreading misinformation and outright lies on social media. But I may never know. I will continue to reach out to her, to send her pictures of her granddaughters, and to let her know that she is more to me than her vaccination status – however crazy I privately think her decision not to be vaccinated is. I don't think my mother – or Maureen, or Noela, or Judy – pose an unacceptable threat to society.

But I do think that people like them could be further isolated and radicalised if they are unnecessarily excluded from society.

It's unclear whether truck protests and convoys are a blip on the political landscape or a movement that's here to stay. We don't know whether tensions will simmer down if mandates are abandoned, or if they will boil over once more should a new variant necessitate additional control measures in the future. A diverse aggregation of groups have united, ostensibly around the issue of mandatory vaccination. They all tapped into a wellspring of distrust – in government, in politicians, and in mainstream media. The 'them vs us' rhetoric of populist politicians found a natural affinity with people whose lives – and their hardships – have reinforced a belief that institutions do not have their best interests in mind.

Opposition to vaccination is a niche political position. But niche political parties can gain real political clout. In 2013, Ricky Muir, running for the Australian Motoring Enthusiasts Party, won a federal senate seat with just 0.51 per cent of the primary vote. Populist anti-elite and anti-government parties may well attract an even larger support base by hitching their wagon to the anti-vax cause. People who started out with questions about a brand new vaccine against a virus they saw as no threat could be – inadvertently or not – bolstering support for a populist vote, which, in other contexts, has led to divisive leaders like Trump and further erosion of trust in government institutions and democratic processes.

For those who followed their antipathy towards vaccines to the darker corners of the internet, ushered along by conspiracy-minded groups, Hornsey offered a glimmer of hope. He told me that in his data, conspiracy thinking and vaccine refusal don't always go hand in hand. 'In my data, the link between being a conspiracy theorist and being anti-vax sort of breaks if the people around you are pro-vax,' he told me. The biggest concern is when people fall into communities, and then isolate themselves from the mainstream. That's when they convince themselves that vaccine refusal is the norm.

Whether we like it or not, anti-vax activists are here to stay. As long as there have been vaccines, there have been people protesting them. Leask argues that the best way to deal with them is to deny them oxygen. Equating all of the unvaxxed in our community with the worst of the anti-vax activists lends the activists credence. It gives them oxygen. It swells their numbers and makes their niche activism appear more popular than it really is. But we shouldn't underestimate the number of people who see misinformation for what it is, who trust the government, trust scientists, trust their doctors and the health system that keeps them healthy, Lewandowsky told me. We can't force others to trust in institutions on our word, but we can listen and empathise with the genuinely held concerns of those in our orbit who have doubts, ensuring that we are not pushing them further into the hands of the anti-vax community. In our conversations, we can all be a clump of solid earth in the bulwark against disillusionment and isolation.

COVID-19 has become an ever-present part of our lives, and will likely continue to wax and wane with the seasons, occasionally alarming authorities into taking extra precautions depending on how infectious or deadly the variant *du jour* is. New viruses, bursting forth from bat caves in Asia, or pig and poultry farms in North America, will test our mettle once again. Countries that fared relatively well during the COVID-19 pandemic had well-resourced public health infrastructure and steadfast community trust in their institutions. The US, judged to be among the best prepared for a pandemic by the Global Health Security Index, serves as a stark reminder that even a country with formidable medical and scientific expertise at its disposal is no match for a nation divided, and whose trust in government and public health institutions has crumbled.

Waxing and waning with the viruses that plague us will be the anti-vax activists and conspiracy theorists, desperate to capture our fearful attention and have us buy into their worldview. This pandemic will continue to surprise us.

Then the next will be upon us. The way in which we communicate with each other, how we show concern for each other's concerns, has the power to quell or exacerbate the trust we have in the media, in our experts, in our office bearers and in each other. Not just in the midst of crisis, but always.

ACKNOWLEDGEMENTS

Writing this book has felt like being sucked into an immense and swirling whirlwind. Protests erupted and dissipated, COVID-19 case numbers surged, fell, then surged again, and policy settings around the world shifted day by day as I reported and wrote. I would not have been able to draw together the stories and opinions and research – let alone my own thoughts – without the immense support and assistance of people along the way.

Vaccines have become a source of tension and resentment throughout the community, and it takes courage to speak openly and honestly in this climate. I am therefore incredibly grateful to the people who lent me their time and shared their personal stories with me. Several people I interviewed – a participant in a vaccine trial, a mother who is unvaxxed, a GP who has administered thousands of vaccine doses to patients – asked to remain anonymous. Others – including Judy, Maureen, Noela and Mel – I have referred to by first name only, to protect their privacy.

I am indebted to the incredible social scientists and researchers who try to understand why we do what we do. Thanks to Julie Leask and Katie Attwell for sharing their wealth of knowledge about vaccination attitudes and how they have shifted over time. Matthew Hornsey, Mathew Marques, Aleksandra Cichocka, Karen Douglas and Stephan Lewandowsky helped me to untangle the connections between vaccine refusal, science denial and belief in conspiracies.

Catherine Bennett's astute analysis of the pandemic's ups and downs helped me to connect the raw numbers of the pandemic with the levers that governments pull to control them. I was grateful for her help at the start of my reporting, and again when Omicron meant that the sands beneath my feet had shifted. Thanks also to Jim Buttery for answering my niggly vaccine questions, to Tony Scott for taking me through the highs and lows of vaccination attitudes over the past two-and-a-half years, and to Dominic Wilkinson for providing me with the ethicist's view on vaccine mandates.

Thank you also to Adam Gibson, for speaking with me about Parents With Questions, and to Isaac Golden, who spoke with me about his alternative health advocacy work. Thanks to Mike Freelander, who spoke to me about vaccine misinformation in politics.

There are many others not mentioned in the book, whose stories have influenced my thinking about vaccination in the era of COVID-19. Close friends who remain unvaccinated, people whose brothers or sisters have become estranged. All shaped my understanding about the mood of the nation on this divisive topic.

I'd like to thank Arwen Summers and Peter Fray for presenting me with such an exciting and rewarding opportunity. From early sketches to deadline – and beyond – they provided smart and insightful feedback on my work, making it stronger at every step. Arwen's encouragement, in particular, propelled me to keep writing when the gremlins of doubt nagged. Thanks also to John Mapps, Anna Collett, Kasi Collins and others whose behind-the-scenes work made the book possible. And to Josh Durham, for his fabulous cover design.

I'd like to thank my partner Brad – for his kid wrangling and his tolerance of my shirtiness, and his continuing support of my career. My daughters also deserve thanks, for allowing me to shoo them out of my office so many times over the past couple of months. They've displayed more patience than I should have expected from their seven- and four-year-old selves. Massive thanks also to my wonderful friend and fellow traveller Viki Cramer, who was at the end of the phone whenever I needed her.

Finally, I'd like to thank my mother, whose eternal scepticism has both torn us apart and influenced my own unending search for answers.

NOTES

1. Katie Attwell, Adam Hannah and Julie Leask, 'COVID-19: talk of "vaccine hesitancy" lets governments off the hook', *Nature*, 22 February 2022, https://www.nature.com/articles/d41586-022-00495-8
2. Frank Beard, Brynley Hull, Julie Leask, Aditi Dey and Peter McIntyre, 'Trends and patterns in vaccination objection, Australia, 2002–2013', *Medical Journal of Australia*, 18 April 2016, https://doi.org/10.5694/mja15.01226
3. WHO, 'Ten threats to global health in 2019', https://www.who.int/news-room/spotlight/ten-threats-to-global-health-in-2019
4. Transparency International Australia, 'Global Corruption Ranking', https://transparency.org.au/global-ranking/
5. Matthew J. Hornsey, Emily A. Harris and Kelly S. Fielding, 'The psychological roots of anti-vaccination attitudes: a 24-nation investigation', *Health Psychology*, 37(4), 2018, https://doi.org/10.1037/hea0000586

6   Reset Australia, *Anti-vaccination & vaccine hesitant narratives intensify in Australian Facebook Groups*, 17 May 2021, https://au.reset.tech/uploads/resetaustralia_social-listening_report_100521-1.pdf

7   'Is Facebook "killing us"? A new study investigates', Northwestern Now, 29 July 2021, https://news.northwestern.edu/stories/2021/07/is-facebook-killing-us-a-new-study-investigates/

8   Apoorva Mandavilli, 'The C.D.C. isn't publishing large portions of the Covid data it collects', *New York Times*, 21 February 2021, https://www.nytimes.com/2022/02/20/health/covid-cdc-data.html

9   Asami Yagi, Yutaka Ueda, Sayaka Ikeda et al., 'The looming health hazard: A wave of HPV-related cancers in Japan is becoming a reality due to the continued suspension of the governmental recommendation of HPV vaccine', *The Lancet*, 12 December 2021, https://doi.org/10.1016/j.lanwpc.2021.100327

10 Center for Countering Digital Hate, *The Disinformation Dozen: Why platforms must act on twelve leading online anti-vaxxers*, May 2021, https://www.counterhate.com/disinformationdozen

11 Dan Milmo, 'Anti-vaxxers making "at least $2.5m" a year from publishing on Substack', *Guardian*, 27 January 2022, https://www.theguardian.com/technology/2022/jan/27/anti-vaxxers-making-at-least-25m-a-year-from-publishing-on-substack

12 William White, *The Story of a Great Delusion in a Series of Matter-of-Fact Chapters*, Allen, London, 1885, p. 595.

13 ABS, 'COVID-19 mortality in Australia', 15 February 2022, https://www.abs.gov.au/articles/covid-19-mortality-australia#key-statistics

14 Charlotte Ward and David Voas, 'The emergence of conspirituality', *Journal of Contemporary Religion*, 26, 2011, https://doi.org/10.1080/13537903.2011.539846

15 Alexander Grab, 'Smallpox vaccination in Napoleonic Italy (1800–1814)', *Napoleonica La Revue*, 30(3), 2017, https://doi.org/10.3917/napo.030.0038

16 Centers for Disease Control and Prevention, 'Rates of COVID-19 cases and deaths by vaccination status', https://covid.cdc.gov/covid-data-tracker/#rates-by-vaccine-status

17 Joe Ondrak and Jordan Wildon, 'Worldwide anti-lockdown protests organized by German cell', Logically, 14 May 2021, https://www.logically.ai/articles/anti-lockdown-protests-organized-by-german-cell

18 Christopher Knaus and Michael McGowan, 'Who's behind Australia's anti-lockdown protests? The German conspiracy group driving marches', *Guardian*, 27 July 2021, https://www.theguardian.com/australia-news/2021/jul/27/who-behind-australia-anti-covid-lockdown-protest-march-rallies-sydney-melbourne-far-right-and-german-conspiracy-groups-driving-protests

19 Emily Berger, 'More children are self-harming since the start of the pandemic', *The Conversation*, 8 September 2021, https://theconversation.com/more-children-are-self-harming-since-the-start-of-the-pandemic-heres-what-parents-and-teachers-can-do-to-help-167436

20 Helen Rusak, '63.5% of Australia's performing artists reported worsening mental health during COVID', *The Conversation*, 19 January 2022, https://theconversation.com/63-5-of-australias-performing-artists-reported-worsening-mental-health-during-covid-174610

21 Katharine Murphy, 'Guardian Essential poll: majority of Australians support vaccine mandates', *Guardian*, 14 September 2021, https://www.theguardian.com/australia-news/2021/sep/14/guardian-essential-poll-majority-of-australians-support-vaccine-mandates
22 Eleonore Batteux, Avri Bilovich, Samuel G.B. Johnson and David Tuckett, 'The negative consequences of failing to communicate uncertainties during a pandemic: The case of COVID-19 vaccines', medRxiv, 1 March 2021, https://www.medrxiv.org/content/10.1101/2021.02.28.21252616v1.full